# Geriatric Pain Management

*Editor*

M. CARRINGTON REID

# CLINICS IN GERIATRIC MEDICINE

www.geriatric.theclinics.com

November 2016 • Volume 32 • Number 4

**ELSEVIER**

1600 John F. Kennedy Boulevard • Suite 1800 • Philadelphia, Pennsylvania, 19103-2899

http://www.theclinics.com

**CLINICS IN GERIATRIC MEDICINE Volume 32, Number 4**
**November 2016 ISSN 0749–0690, ISBN-13: 978-0-323-47683-6**

Editor: Jessica McCool
Developmental Editor: Colleen Viola

*Clinics in Geriatric Medicine* (ISSN 0749-0690) is published quarterly by Elsevier Inc., 360 Park Avenue South, New York, NY 10010-1710. Months of issue are February, May, August, and November. Business and Editorial Offices: 1600 John F. Kennedy Blvd., Suite 1800, Philadelphia, PA 191023-2899. Periodicals postage paid at New York, NY, and additional mailing offices. Subscription prices are $265.00 per year (US individuals), $557.00 per year (US institutions), $100.00 per year (US student/resident), $370.00 per year (Canadian individuals), $706.00 per year (Canadian institutions), $195.00 per year (Canadian student/resident), $390.00 per year (international individuals), $706.00 per year (international institutions), and $195.00 per year (international student/resident). Foreign air speed delivery is included in all *Clinics* subscription prices. All prices are subject to change without notice. POSTMASTER: Send address changes to *Clinics in Geriatric Medicine*, Elsevier Health Sciences Division, Subscription Customer Service, 3251 Riverport Lane, Maryland Heights, MO 63043. **Telephone: 1-800-654-2452 (U.S. and Canada); 314-447-8871 (outside U.S. and Canada). Fax: 314-447-8029. E-mail:** journalscustomerservice-usa@elsevier. com **(for print support) or** journalsonlinesupport-usa@elsevier.com **(for online support).**

*Reprints.* For copies of 100 or more, of articles in this publication, please contact the Commercial Reprints Department, Elsevier Inc., 360 Park Avenue South, New York, New York 10010-1710. Tel.: 212-633-3874; Fax: 212-633-3820, E-mail: reprints@elsevier.com.

*Clinics in Geriatric Medicine* is covered in *MEDLINE/PubMed (Index Medicus), EMBASE/Excerpta Medica, Current Contents/Clinical Medicine (CC/CM),* and the *Cumulative Index to Nursing & Allied Health Literature.*

# Contributors

## EDITOR

**M. CARRINGTON REID, MD, PhD**
Director, Translational Research Institute on Pain in Later Life; Associate Professor of
Medicine, Division of Geriatrics and Palliative Medicine, Weill Cornell Medicine, New York,
New York

## AUTHORS

**PRIN X. AMORAPANTH, MD, PhD**
Clinical Instructor and Research Faculty, Department of Rehabilitation, Rusk
Rehabilitation at New York University Langone Medical Center, New York, New York

**KATHERINE BEISSNER, PT, PhD**
Department of Physical Therapy Education, SUNY Upstate Medical University, Syracuse,
New York

**STAJA Q. BOOKER, MS, RN, PhD(c)**
Nursing Doctoral Candidate, The University of Iowa, College of Nursing, Iowa City, Iowa

**AMBER K. BROOKS, MD**
Assistant Professor, Department of Anesthesiology, Wake Forest School of Medicine,
Winston-Salem, North Carolina

**RACHAEL ELIZABETH DOCKING, PhD, MA (Hons)**
Faculty of Health, Social Care and Education; Research Fellow, Anglia Ruskin
University-London, Chelmsford, Essex, United Kingdom; Senior Evidence Manager,
Centre for Ageing Better, London, United Kingdom

**NAKIA A. DUNCAN, PharmD**
Assistant Professor, Texas Tech University Health Sciences Center School of Pharmacy,
Dallas, Texas

**CHRISTOPHER ECCLESTON, PhD**
Centre for Pain Research, The University of Bath, Bath, United Kingdom

**RHIANNON TERRI EDWARDS, MSc**
Centre for Pain Research, The University of Bath, Bath, United Kingdom

**TERRI FRIED, MD**
Professor of Medicine (Geriatrics), Department of Internal Medicine, Yale School of
Medicine, New Haven, Connecticut; Clinical Epidemiology Unit, Geriatrics and Extended
Care, Department of Internal Medicine (Geriatrics), Veterans Affairs Connecticut
Healthcare System, West Haven, Connecticut

**WALID F. GELLAD, MD, MPH**
Physician Researcher, Center for Health Equity Research and Promotion, Veterans Affairs Pittsburgh Healthcare System, University of Pittsburgh; Associate Professor, Division of General Medicine, Department of Medicine, University of Pittsburgh School of Medicine, Pittsburgh, Pennsylvania

**STEPHEN J. GIBSON, PhD, MAPsS**
Clinical Division, National Ageing Research Institute, Parkville, Victoria, Australia

**JOSEPH T. HANLON, PharmD, MS**
Health Scientist; Professor of Geriatric Medicine, Pharmacy, and Epidemiology, Center for Health Equity Research and Promotion, Geriatric Research Education and Clinical Center, Veterans Affairs Pittsburgh Healthcare System, University of Pittsburgh, Pittsburgh, Pennsylvania

**KEELA A. HERR, RN, PhD, FAAN, AGSF**
Professor and Associate Dean for Faculty, The University of Iowa, College of Nursing, Iowa City, Iowa

**SHARON KAASALAINEN, RN, PhD**
Associate Professor, School of Nursing, McMaster University, Hamilton, Ontario, Canada

**EDMUND KEOGH, PhD**
Centre for Pain Research, The University of Bath, Bath, United Kingdom

**SEAN LAUBENSTEIN, DPT**
Chittenango Physical Therapy, Chittenango, New York

**UNA E. MAKRIS, MD, MSc**
Assistant Professor, Division of Rheumatic Diseases, Department of Internal Medicine, Veterans Affairs North Texas Health Care System, UT Southwestern Medical Center, Dallas, Texas

**ZACHARY A. MARCUM, PharmD, PhD**
Assistant Professor, Department of Pharmacy, University of Washington School of Pharmacy, Seattle, Washington

**JENNIFER GREENE NAPLES, PharmD**
Post-doctoral Geriatrics Pharmacotherapy Fellow, Division of Geriatrics & Gerontology, Department of Medicine, University of Pittsburgh School of Medicine, University of Pittsburgh, Pittsburgh, Pennsylvania

**VEERAWAT PHONGTANKUEL, MD**
Instructor in Medicine, Division of Geriatrics and Palliative Medicine, Department of Medicine, Weill Cornell Medicine, New York, New York

**KARL PILLEMER, PhD**
Hazel E. Reed Professor, Department of Human Development; Professor of Gerontology in Medicine, Weill Cornell Medicine; Director of the Bronfenbrenner Center for Translational Research, College of Human Ecology, Cornell University, Ithaca, New York

**M. CARRINGTON REID, MD, PhD**
Director, Translational Research Institute on Pain in Later Life; Associate Professor of Medicine, Division of Geriatrics and Palliative Medicine, Weill Cornell Medicine, New York, New York

**CATHERINE RIFFIN, PhD**
Post-doctoral Fellow in Medicine (Geriatrics), Department of Internal Medicine, Yale School of Medicine, New Haven, Connecticut

**STEVEN M. SAVVAS, PhD**
Clinical Division, National Ageing Research Institute, Parkville, Victoria, Australia

**EUGENIA L. SIEGLER, MD**
Professor of Clinical Medicine and Mason Adams Professor of Geriatric Medicine, Division of Geriatrics and Palliative Medicine, Department of Medicine, Weill Cornell Medicine, New York, New York

**ABBY TABOR, PhD**
Centre for Pain Research, The University of Bath, Bath, United Kingdom

**MERCY A. UDOJI, MD, CMQ**
Department of Anesthesiology, Interventional Pain Management, Veterans Affairs Medical Center, Atlanta, Georgia

**ABIGAIL WICKSON-GRIFFITHS, RN, PhD**
Assistant Professor, Faculty of Nursing, University of Regina, Regina, Saskatchewan, Canada

# Contents

Epidemiological data suggests that the prevalence of musculoskeletal and neuropathic pain increases with age until at least late mid-life, though the pattern is somewhat unclear beyond this point. And though the prevalence of some types of pain may peak in late midlife, pain is still a substantial and common complaint even in the oldest age groups. This article provides an overview of later-life pain and includes a brief review of its epidemiology, describes commonly encountered barriers to its management, and discusses guidelines and recommended approaches to its assessment and management.

The World Health Organization, one of the leading authorities on pain management, stressed the need for further guidelines to help manage pain in patients with chronic disease. In light of the impact of pain on morbidity and quality of life, this article summarizes current knowledge about pain experienced by older adults in 3 advanced non–cancer-related chronic diseases (ie, congestive heart failure, end-stage renal disease, and stroke) in which pain is common but not typically a primary focus of disease management. This article examines the data on the prevalence of pain, co-occurring symptoms, and challenges in managing pain in these conditions.

This article provides an overview of the literature describing the effects of geriatric patients' pain on family members' relationships, psychological well-being, and physical health. The theoretic mechanisms that underlie the association between patients' pain and family members' outcomes are outlined, and studies describing these mechanisms are summarized. Limitations to the current literature are discussed, and key recommendations for future research and practice are presented.

Pain in aging adults is a global health problem requiring a proactive and consistent assessment approach. Pain assessment is critical to detecting pain and developing a collaborative and adaptive pain management plan. Getting health providers to assess and measure pain even in older adults who are communicative and can self-report remains a challenge.

Self-report is the best method for identifying pain. Using a validated pain assessment scale is key to evaluate pain intensity. This article discusses techniques to obtain self-report and describe appropriate self-report pain tools for a focused pain assessment and reassessment in adults in later life.

An interdisciplinary approach to managing pain has been widely used in managing specific pain conditions (eg, lower back and fibromyalgia) but not reviewed specifically for older adults. Interdisciplinary approaches have been used in primary, residential long-term, and acute care settings, where a variety of health care professionals work on pain teams to manage pain in older adults. Given the multidimensional nature of pain in older adults, interdisciplinary approaches to managing pain are recommended in practice. This article reviews the rationale supporting an interdisciplinary approach to managing pain in older adults and summarizes studies that have evaluated this approach.

Pharmacologic management of chronic pain in older adults is one component of the multimodal, interdisciplinary management of this complex condition. In this article, we summarize several of the key barriers to effective pharmacologic management in older adults and review the existing (albeit limited) evidence for its effectiveness and safety, especially in a medically complex population with multimorbidity. This review covers topical formulations, acetaminophen, oral nonsteroidal antiinflammatory drugs, and adjuvant therapies. The article concludes with a suggested approach to managing chronic pain in the older patient, incorporating goals and expectations for treatment as well as careful monitoring of medication adjustments.

When possible, chronic noncancer pain (CNCP) in older adults should be managed by nonpharmacologic modalities in conjunction with nonopioid analgesics. If moderate-to-severe pain persists despite these approaches, however, nonparenteral opioids may be considered as adjunctive therapy. This article reviews the epidemiology of opioid use and their effectiveness for CNCP in older adults and summarizes important age-related changes in opioid pharmacokinetics and pharmacodynamics that increase the risks of adverse effects in the elderly. Finally, to assist clinicians with selecting appropriate therapy, the article concludes with an evidence-based approach to optimize opioid prescribing in older adults with CNCP.

Exercise is often recommended for older adults with pain, but pain itself is often a barrier to increased activity. This article reviews the evidence on the impact of various forms of exercise and related movement therapies on older adults with pain problems. The literature is reviewed with respect to published guidelines. When prescribing exercise, it is important to consider appropriate intensity, type, and duration of exercise as well as incorporating a plan for progression. Strategies to ensure adherence to exercise programs are also important.

A psychological model of coping with the demands of aging is outlined. Chronic pain is conceptualized as a challenge to normal aging, because it threatens identity, risks affective disorder (depression), and interferes with action. The sparse evidence for psychological interventions is reviewed, and a case is made for the types of interventions that should be developed to address the specific presentation of geriatric pain management.

Chronic pain in older patients is often treated with pain medications, physical rehabilitation, interventional pain management, and/or psychological interventions. The administration of pain medications is the most common form of chronic pain treatment. Physiologic changes in older adults make them more susceptible to the potential side effects of oral pain medications, especially opioids. Interventional pain management offers an alternative treatment option. This article reviews some of the interventional techniques used to treat the most common sites of pain in older adults: back, knee, and hip.

This article provides a brief overview of the challenges and opportunities of new technologies in the area of geriatric pain management. It also reviews emerging evidence to demonstrate the role technology may play in improving and advancing assessment and management of pain in older adults.

Clinicians are often challenged to find targets for intervention in older adults with chronic pain. This article highlights 3 targets clinicians should consider when formulating their multimodal treatment plans to include older patients' attitudes and beliefs about pain and pain treatments, expectations regarding treatment outcomes, and pleasurable activity pursuits.

# CLINICS IN GERIATRIC MEDICINE

# Preface

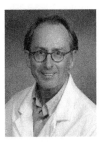

M. Carrington Reid, MD, PhD
*Editor*

Later life pain is a worldwide problem that adversely affects older adults in both developed and developing countries. It is associated with substantial disability that occurs by way of reduced mobility, activity avoidance, falls, depression and anxiety, and social isolation. The negative effects of pain extend well beyond the patient, often disrupting both family and social relationships. It is also important to note that later life pain poses a significant economic burden at a societal level. One recent analysis found that the annual cost of pain in the United States was nearly 30% higher than the costs of cancer and diabetes combined.[1] Prevalence rates for pain will likely increase as the population ages, thereby increasing its public health impact. Given the scope and magnitude of the problem, it is now widely recognized that health care providers must develop competencies to assess and manage pain in their older patients.

This issue of *Clinics in Geriatric Medicine* seeks to help readers develop core competencies in managing pain by providing information about key topics in geriatric pain management. The articles have been written by experts in the field and provide practical up-to-date information on assessment and management approaches as well as emerging topics that readers should find useful. Readers will learn about the epidemiology of common pain disorders to include specific pain problems that occur commonly in older adults with chronic illness. Evidence-based assessment approaches are presented that are appropriate for use in a busy office setting. Pharmacotherapies are summarized to include the role of opioid medications for older patients whose pain cannot be effectively controlled with other modalities. Specific nonpharmacologic strategies are covered to include exercise and movement-based modalities as well as psychological approaches that should be core components of any treatment plan. Readers will also learn about the evidence underlying specific interventional approaches (eg, epidural injections), the growing role of technologies (eg, mobile health) in pain care, and the impact of an older adult's pain on family members. Finally, underutilized targets for intervention are presented to include patients' beliefs about pain, their expectations regarding treatment outcomes, and the important role of pleasant activity scheduling. A common theme that runs throughout the articles is the need for formulating multimodal treatment approaches that include both drug and nondrug modalities and interdisciplinary input when possible. Finally, although

Clin Geriatr Med 32 (2016) xi–xii
http://dx.doi.org/10.1016/j.cger.2016.08.011
0749-0690/16/© 2016 Published by Elsevier Inc.

the evidence base about how best to manage pain in the older adult continues to grow, important knowledge gaps remain and are presented in the articles.

I hope that readers will gain practical knowledge as a result of reading these articles. It is my sincerest hope, however, that readers apply this knowledge in practice, ultimately leading to improved pain care and care outcomes in this growing population of patients.

M. Carrington Reid, MD, PhD
Division of Geriatrics and Palliative Medicine
Weill Cornell Medical College
New York, NY 10065, USA

E-mail address:
mcr2004@med.cornell.edu

**REFERENCE**

1. Gaskin DJ, Richard P. The economic costs of pain in the United States. J Pain 2012;13(8):715–24.

# Overview of Pain Management in Older Adults

Steven M. Savvas, PhD*, Stephen J. Gibson, PhD, MAPsS

## KEYWORDS

• Pain • Pain management • Older • Prevalence • Barriers • Cognitive impairment

## KEY POINTS

- Pain in older people is common. Whether pain prevalence increases, decreases, or plateaus with advancing age may be related to the type of pain.
- Considerable barriers to pain management exist and include attitudes (patient and health provider), communication, effect of age on pharmacokinetics, and comorbidities.
- A broad approach to pain management for older people is recommended and is similar to that used in younger cohorts: pain identification and assessment, pain management with pharmacologic and nonpharmacologic approaches, and evaluation of side effects.

## INTRODUCTION

The population is aging. Globally more than 900 million people are 60 years of age or older, and this group is growing at a rate of more than 3% per year.[1] More than 20% of the population in Europe and North America are currently more than 60 years of age, and projections estimate that most major regions in the world will have at least a quarter of their population more than 60 years old by 2050. This shift in demographics has caused a proliferation of research in older persons, addressing the considerable gaps that previously existed. Pain in older people has likewise seen considerable work this century,[2] with substantial recent progress in pain and dementia.

Pain is a sufficiently different experience for older adults compared with younger cohorts, in part because of key differences between these groups, such as physiologic differences, pain perception, attitudes about pain, coping ability, and social support/context.[3] Despite these differences, pain management in older people is similar to approaches used in younger cohorts: identify and assess for pain, manage pain with a

Disclosures: S.M. Savvas has nothing to disclose. Professor S.J. Gibson is on an education bureau with Pfizer Pty Ltd and is on an advisory board for BioCSL Pty Ltd.
Clinical Division, National Ageing Research Institute, 34-48 Poplar Road, Parkville, Victoria 3052, Australia
* Corresponding author.
E-mail address: s.savvas@nari.unimelb.edu.au

Clin Geriatr Med 32 (2016) 635–650
http://dx.doi.org/10.1016/j.cger.2016.06.005
0749-0690/16/© 2016 Elsevier Inc. All rights reserved.

geriatric.theclinics.com

multimodal approach using pharmacologic and nonpharmacologic treatments, and evaluate side effects and benefits of treatment. However, special consideration is needed in older adults, who often have more comorbidity, are prescribed more medications, experience more serious drug side effects, have significantly more sensory and cognitive impairments, and have differing attitudes to disablement and pain management goals (often attributable to common circumstances, such as retirement). These differences affect general approaches when managing pain in older adults.

This article provides an overview of later-life pain and includes a brief review of its epidemiology, describes commonly encountered barriers to its management, and discusses guidelines and recommended approaches to both its assessment and management.

## EPIDEMIOLOGY

Pain prevalence is difficult to estimate in older persons. Self-reported pain is the gold standard and although this acknowledges that pain is subjective and personal, self-report is also subject to personal biases stemming from personality and generational traits (eg, stoicism), culture, and especially age-related impairments such as sensory loss and cognitive impairment. Prevalence reports differ from country to country, with some variability caused by the demographics of the populations being investigated, the setting (eg, community, long-term care, hospital), pain definition (eg, acute, chronic, current pain, >3 months, lifetime), the type and site of pain, pain management approaches used, and differences in research methods. For all these reasons, pain prevalence reporting needs specificity when making comparisons.

Pain prevalence estimates differ greatly between countries, although chronic pain prevalence studies are lacking in many developing countries, especially those with limited resources.[4] A review of chronic pain[5] reported significantly high prevalence for persons aged 66 years or older in developing countries (South Africa, China, Americas, Ukraine, Nigeria, and Lebanon) compared with the developed countries of western Europe, North America, Japan, and New Zealand. Furthermore, there is considerable variation among developing countries, with a recent study[6] that used standardized national data showing low back pain prevalence ranging from a low of 22% (China) to a high of 55.7% (Russian Federation). Disease prevalence estimates of conditions that are typically pain promoting further distinguish the differences between developed and developing countries, although they may also indicate that the prevalence of certain conditions is higher in developed countries. For example, osteoarthritis of the knee is more prevalent in many developed countries (especially in North America, Europe, Australia, Japan, and New Zealand) compared with the western pacific region, south east Asia, Africa, and countries in the eastern Mediterranean.[7] Furthermore, this gap widens for the older age cohorts. However, there are few epidemiologic studies on other musculoskeletal disorders, such as rheumatoid arthritis, and no research data for many African countries. A recent review suggests that a crude prevalence of rheumatoid arthritis in Africa is substantially lower compared with North America and Europe.[8–10]

Living situation (ie, residing in a community vs residential/long-term care setting) seems to be a useful demarcation when reviewing pain prevalence. Although only a few older adults reside in long-term care facilities, this cohort is representative of a group that conceivably experiences significant barriers in pain management. For example, most patients in long-term care have cognitive impairment and multiple comorbidities, and therefore prevalence figures for this group represent a useful upper limit of pain in older adults. Among community-dwelling older adults, pain prevalence estimates of current pain (ie, pain described as "in the moment") vary from 20% to 46%.[11,12] Chronic pain in the community also shows a comparable lower limit in prevalence, with an upper limit ranging from 25% to 76% prevalence,[11,13–19] although the definition of chronic pain is inconsistent. In contrast, the prevalence of current pain in long-term aged care settings is higher still, from 28% to 73%,[20–25] and can be very high for chronic pain, with prevalence estimates up to 93%.[21,25,26]

## Pain and Advancing Age

The role of advancing age in pain prevalence is not clear and an overall pattern is hard to discern. A review of 39 studies[27] suggests 4 patterns regarding how pain prevalence changes with age: (1) increases with age, (2) increases until 75 to 85 years old and then decreases (although other studies suggest prevalence peaks much earlier; from 50–65 years of age), (3) decreases, or (4) no difference with age. Most of the articles reviewed were related to either unspecified pain type or musculoskeletal pain. Reconciling the conflicting patterns is difficult, although grouping these patterns by type of pain (as is done later) may be insightful.

Research on the prevalence of neuropathic pain is equivocal; one study showed that neuropathic pain continues to increase with age,[28] although a large postal survey reported that chronic daily pain with neuropathic characteristics increased until 50 to 64 years old, then plateaued at about 9% prevalence.[29] Musculoskeletal pain may also peak at midlife.[30,31] A systematic review on the prevalence of low back pain[32] concluded from 6 studies that chronic lower back pain prevalence is lowest in younger adults (20–30 years), increases until around 50 to 60 years old, and then is stable or decreases. However, a systematic literature review on back and neck pain[33] reported scant evidence of increased back pain prevalence in people less than 60 years old versus more than 60 years old, but concluded that there was some evidence that back pain prevalence generally declines in the oldest old. Another systematic review[34] suggested significant heterogeneity in good-quality back pain prevalence studies, with between 5 and 13 studies able to be characterized into one of the 4 patterns described previously. The review concluded that pain severity may have a substantial effect on the relationship between back pain and advancing age, with severe back pain prevalence increasing with age, whereas the prevalence pattern for benign and mixed back pain seems to increase with advancing age, peaks at 50 to 60 years old, and then declines. **Fig. 1** presents data from several select studies and shows the variability in pain prevalence estimates for back-related and neck-related pain across the life span.

Myocardial infarction–related pain may decrease[35] with age, as may migraine and severe headaches. A review[36] of US National Health Survey data shows that the prevalence of severe headache or migraine is highest in people aged 18 to 54 years (around 19%), but decreases for those 65 to 74 years old (9.5%) and 75 years old and older (6.1%). There is also some evidence that cancer pain prevalence decreases with age because pain symptom prevalence was higher patients with advanced cancer aged less than 65 years (88%) than more than 65 years (80%), although a more recent study showed no difference in pain symptom prevalence between those less than 60 years old, from 60 to 69 years, and greater than or equal to 70 years old.[37] **Fig. 2** shows pain prevalence estimates across the life span for a range of pain conditions from a select number of studies.

## Type and Sites of Pain

Studies suggest that the following are the most common pain complaints in older people: osteoarthritic back/neck pain (a complaint voiced by about 65% of older adults),

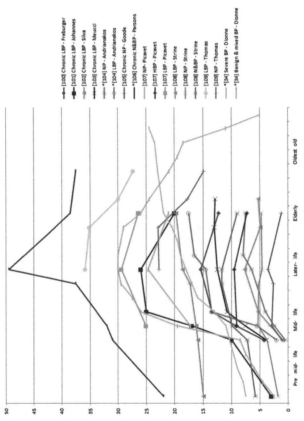

**Fig. 1.** Pain prevalence across the life span for back-related and neck-related pain (select studies). Age groups are premidlife (approximately <25 years old), midlife (approximately 30–50 years old), later life (approximately 50–65 years old), elderly (approximately 65–80 years old), and oldest old (approximately ≥80 years old). Numbers in bracket indicate reference numbers; asterisks indicate estimated values. BP, back pain; HBP, higher back pain; LBP, lower back pain; N&BP, neck and back pain; NP, neck pain. *Data from* Refs.[34,100–109]

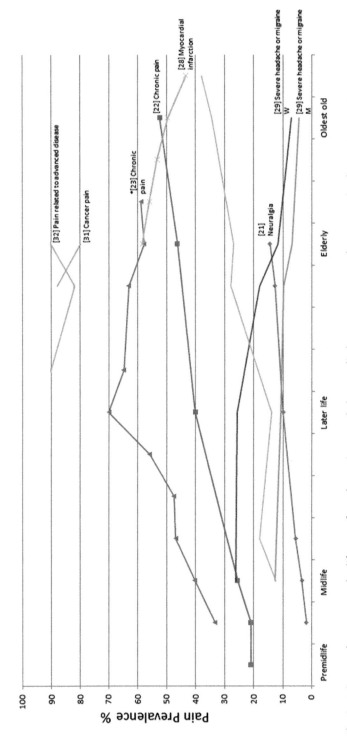

**Fig. 2.** Pain prevalence across the life span for other pain types (select studies). Age groups are the same as in **Fig. 1**. M, men; W, women.

musculoskeletal pain (about 40%), peripheral neuropathic pain (about 35%), and chronic joint pain (15%–25%).[38–40] A review of 22 studies[27] that reported pain at different sites found that back pain, leg/knee/hip, and other joints were the 3 most common locations for pain. A larger systematic review[41] of the prevalence of musculoskeletal conditions in older people in developed countries showed similar but lower prevalence rates, with back pain (neck, midback, or lower back) as the most commonly reported conditions (29%), followed by osteoporosis and osteoarthritis (17%), rheumatoid arthritis (8%), ankle/foot pain (8%), knee pain (6%), hip pain (5%), shoulder pain (5%), hand/wrist pain (3%), and elbow pain (3%). A nationally representative sample of American adults aged 65 to 69 years showed back (30.4%), knee (25.0%), and shoulder (20.9%) were the most prevalent sites of pain, with this pattern remaining little changed with older cohorts (eg, for the oldest cohort of 90 years or older, the most prevalent sites were back [32.0%], knee [28.5%], and shoulder [22.4%]).[42] How pain type is categorized often varies between studies and there is sometimes no clear demarcation between the site of pain and the type of pain. However, it is clear that the back and joints are the leading sites for pain in older people.

Of particular interest is the number of sites that a patient reports as painful. Pain in multiple sites is common, with pain reported at 2 or more sites by 40% of people aged 65 years or older.[43,44] Furthermore, musculoskeletal pain that is present with pain in other sites has been shown to be more disabling and severe,[45] and linked with a poorer prognosis with regard to function, mood, and daily activities.[46]

### Risk Factors

Several studies have either inferred risk factors from pain prevalence estimates or have used statistical methods such as logistic regression to identify risk factors for pain in older people. One of the most salient risk factors is gender, with most studies identifying women as more likely to experience pain.[11–19] Several large community cohort European studies suggest roughly a 10-point difference for women compared with men in people more than 75 years old reporting joint pain (UK, 64% of women reported joint pain in at least 1 site vs 49% of men[47]; France, 43% of women reported joint pain vs 36% of men[48]). Although the most prominent risk factor for osteoarthritis is age, partly as a consequence of cumulative exposure to movement of joints and to age-associated biological and anatomic changes, women are both more likely to have osteoarthritis and more likely to have more severe osteoarthritis.[49]

Race/ethnicity is another risk factor and a review of 27 studies conducted in the United States reported higher pain intensity/prevalence[50] and poorer pain management for minority adults 60 years old or older.[50,51] Studies (that included but were not exclusively older adults) in the United Kingdom similarly show differences between different ethnic and minority populations, with both musculoskeletal pain[52] and chronic widespread pain[53] being more prevalent in ethnic minorities. Other risk factors identified for chronic pain include weight and psychological factors such as depressive mood. For example, obesity has been associated with pain severity and experience,[54] with abdominal obesity almost doubling the risk of chronic pain in older adults.[55] Depression has also been strongly associated with chronic pain, both as a consequence of experiencing chronic pain and as a risk factor for the onset of a painful episode.[56]

### Summary

Pain is a significant problem in both community and institutionalized settings, with back and musculoskeletal pain reported most often in older people. Women are also more likely than men to report pain. Pain prevalence may decrease in the oldest old, although pain type is a contributing factor in pain prevalence patterns. However, the data also show that pain in the very old remains a substantial problem. It is therefore essential that pain management in older people is managed well and with an approach that acknowledges the multidimensionality of pain, especially because there are considerable barriers that make treatment challenging.

## BARRIERS TO PAIN MANAGEMENT

Fairly comprehensive guidance on the management of pain in older people[27] has summarized several salient barriers regarding the identification, assessment, and management of pain. Attitudes and beliefs, communications, and changes affecting drug handling and thus pharmacologic pain management were all identified as potential barriers. Other impediments that play a role include polypharmacy, comorbidities, functional limitations, and physical inactivity or inability, as well as systematic barriers in health care systems.

Attitudes to pain in older people may be either beneficial or a barrier. Older people frequently report that pain is to be expected with increasing age. This finding may suggest that older people are better able to cope with chronic pain than younger people. However, misattribution of pain to aging, rather than disease, may also be counterproductive if the patient then believes that pain should be tolerated or cannot be treated, and therefore does not seek medical care.[57,58] Stoicism to pain (enduring pain without complaint) has been highlighted as a trait particular in older people[59] that results in underreporting pain or minimizing its impact. Fear of an unfavorable diagnosis may also explain an older adult's reluctance to report pain, especially because this may signal the progression of an existing illness, or loss of independence.[60]

The pain experience is also strongly influenced by psychological factors. Patients who endorse high levels of pain catastrophizing have been shown to have poorer pain outcomes, and more recent evidence suggests that positive traits, such as optimism/hope, lessen pain perception via reduced levels of pain catastrophizing.[61] Therefore, identifying patients susceptible to pain catastrophizing, pessimism, or hopelessness may be particularly useful when recommending psychological services (such as cognitive behavior interventions). Attitudes among health care professionals may also have a profound effect on the attitudes, beliefs, management, and outcomes for patients with chronic pain. A review[62] showed that many health care providers have strong fear avoidance beliefs, which are associated with strong fear avoidance beliefs in their patients. Therefore, health care providers are instrumental in promoting the formation of attitudes and beliefs that are conducive to better pain treatment outcomes.

Communication is another major barrier to pain management in older adults, with dementia particularly affecting pain treatment. A review of early studies reported a reduced use of analgesics in treating pain in people with dementia,[63] although more recent studies indicate that this trend may have been reversed, with even potential overtreatment.[64,65] The presence of cognitive deficits, especially in memory and language domains, limits the use of pain identification and assessment using self-report. However, self-report may still be meaningful for people with dementia, and research suggests that a high completion rate is possible on at least 1 self-report scale for patients with moderate dementia.[66]

The effect of aging on medications shows several potentially substantial pharmacokinetic changes. Reduced drug absorption and changes in drug distribution, and poorer drug metabolism with reduced drug excretion, are typical in older people.

Compliance with pain medication regimes may be suboptimal, because older patients typically take pain medications less frequently and often at lower than prescribed doses.[67] Concerns over side effects, fear of addiction, and lapses in memory are all contributory factors. Polypharmacy is also a considerable risk in older people, with at least 40% of older patients across a variety of settings (eg, hospital, long-term care) on more than 5 prescribed medications.[68,69] As a result, drug-drug interactions are a particular concern.

## GUIDELINES AND APPROACHES TO PAIN MANAGEMENT

It is not surprising that pain management in older people may be different from that used in younger cohorts, although the broad steps remain similar: pain identification and assessment; pain management, typically using pharmacologic and nonpharmacologic approaches; and ongoing evaluation of side effects and benefits.

### Identification and Assessment of Pain

Comprehensive pain assessment is vital in tailoring an effective pain management strategy. (See Staja Q. Booker and Keela A. Herrs' article, "Assessment and Measurement of Pain in Adults in Later Life," in this issue). Correct diagnosis of the cause of pain better ensures the use of the most effective treatment (as also, the underlying cause of pain may be remediable). When considering any new diagnostic investigation, it is important to note that there may be a high occurrence of incidental disorders and that abnormal findings may be unrelated to any reported pain symptoms.[70] The need for expensive imaging tests should therefore be considered with care. These tests may reassure geriatric patients that the pain is not caused by an underlying serious disorder, but imaging costs are substantial. A recent study suggests that there may also be little value in early diagnostic imaging of older people with back pain, because 12-month outcomes on pain disability were similar to those of patients without early diagnostic imaging.[71] A selective approach to imaging in low back pain is recommended and a recent review[72] suggests that, when red flags are absent (eg, risk factors for cancer/spinal infections, severe neurologic deficits), imaging should be deferred until after an initial 1-month trial of conventional therapy coupled with a lack of improvement.

Several assessment approaches are available to identify and assess the presence of pain and its impact. Self-report scales or observational/behavioral scales may be appropriate as circumstances warrant.[73] Self-report is the gold standard, despite potential attitudinal and other barriers, and the most effective scales are simply worded and easily understood. More complex multidimensional scales may be advantageous to assess other pain-related impacts such as sleep, mood, and function, and this can be important when formulating a treatment plan.

With advancing cognitive limitations, observational scales are increasingly used. Several scales have been developed for use in patients with severe dementia, although none stand out. A key component to observational scales is to note particular behaviors that indicate pain. Common elements in these scales are facial expressions, body language, and vocalizations, although these behaviors may also indicate nonpainful events such as fatigue/exertion. Scales have also been developed to differentiate neuropathic pain from nociceptive pain[74] and may be of use in older adults. If more rigorous and standardized testing is needed then quantitative sensory testing may be of benefit,[75] although these methods are still considered as research tools. Several other scales are also available to assess pain's impact on key domains such as older people's physical[76,77] or psychological function.[78]

## Pain Management

Managing persistent pain is complex, irrespective of age, and several guidelines for managing pain in older people are available.[27,73,79–81] A multimodal approach using pharmacologic and nonpharmacologic therapies is recommended, although the relationship between patient and health care professional is also central to effective treatment.[82,83] Especially vital is the need for mutually agreed and realistic treatment goals, as well as patients having confidence that health care professionals will be available and can provide advice and support.

### Pharmacologic pain treatments

Regardless of age, pharmacologic management of pain is a central tenet. (See Zachary A. Marcum and colleagues' article, "Pharmacotherapies in Geriatric Chronic Pain Management," in this issue). However, because of age-related alterations in drug pharmacokinetics, pain medication recommendations differ for older people. Acetaminophen (paracetamol) is still considered the first-line therapy for pain (especially musculoskeletal-related pain) because of its efficacy and favorable safety profile. Adverse drug effects are rare, although recommended maximum daily doses should not be exceeded (with some suggestion of 800 mg per dose instead of 1000 mg). The use of long-term nonsteroidal antiinflammatory drugs (NSAIDs) needs careful monitoring in older people because of increased associations with gastrointestinal bleeding and ulceration, renal effects, and increased risk of congestive heart failure. NSAIDs may be a more effective treatment than paracetamol for inflammatory pain,[84] but caution is advised[85] because almost a quarter of hospitalizations caused by adverse drug effects in older people have been linked to NSAID use.[86] Some recent American[79] and British[27] geriatric pain guidelines now suggest limited use of oral NSAIDs.

Opioids have shown efficacy for a range of severe chronic pain types[80] (musculoskeletal, cancer, and neuropathic pain), although there is insufficient evidence recommending their use for long-term treatment[87] and opioids are considered as a second-line or third-line therapy for neuropathic pain. A recent review only recommends long-term opioid therapy for older people when other avenues have been exhausted and there are significant impairments in function and daily living.[81] Weak opioids for moderate pain and atypical opioids may also be effective, and have reduced likelihood of side effects such as constipation. In general, side effects of opioids may also need more prophylactic management because chronic constipation is a more serious and recurring problem in many older people. Opioids increase the risk of falls, particularly in the first 2 weeks of use, underscoring the established relationship between pain and falls.[88] Fears of addiction with opioids seem unfounded because studies suggest that the risk of addiction is low in patients without a history of drug dependence.[89,90] Adjuvants may also be appropriate (eg, antidepressants and anticonvulsants), particularly for neuropathic pain. Adverse effects may be considerable when using tricyclics, although there may be fewer anticholinergic adverse effects with a second-generation tricyclic antidepressant.[91]

### Nonpharmacologic pain treatments

Nonpharmacologic therapies, such as physical and psychological therapies, also play a central role in the management of chronic pain in older people. (See Sean Laubenstein and Katherine Beissners' article, "Exercise and Movement-Based Therapies in Geriatric Pain Management," and Christopher Eccleston and colleagues' article, "Psychological Approaches to Coping with Pain in Later Life," in this issue). Physical activity and exercise are viewed as particularly important nonpharmacologic therapies. Alternative movement-based physical therapies (eg, tai chi, yoga) may also be appropriate because these have lower safety concerns for older people, although the evidence base is still not well established. Pain itself is an often-cited barrier that limits activity and impedes the optimal use of physical therapies for older patients with chronic pain. Nonetheless the benefits of physical therapies are clear, with the evidence base showing that, for patients with chronic pain, any type of exercise is better than none,[92] and that activity reduces disability and improves quality of life.[93] However, some caution is warranted with the clinical application of physical activity. Minimizing adverse events such as falls may mean modifying exercise programs and increasing vigilance. Exercise is health promoting but overuse may be pain promoting. Moderate levels of activity are associated with less pain,[94] whereas physical activity levels that are too low are insufficient and levels that are too high are linked with lower back pain.[95]

There is a strong rationale for using psychological therapies for pain management in older patients, because active self-management approaches may be more beneficial in a cohort characterized as passive receivers of health care and generally with an external locus of control.[96] Furthermore, older people are more likely to experience a loss of social support networks through natural attrition, which suggests that the support groups that are part of some psychological therapies may be of particular benefit. Psychological therapies are well received by older adults and can lead to improvements in self-reported pain, although other treatment outcomes (eg, mood, beliefs, disability) are mixed.[97] Due consideration of the treatment goals of older patients is important, because this can be substantially different than for younger cohorts. For example, vocational rehabilitation may no longer be relevant for retirees, whereas social interaction and functional independence in activities of daily living may be of greater priority. Psychological therapies also play a critical role when pain is comorbid with depression. Research suggests that pain, functional impact, and depression interact differently in older people compared with younger cohorts. Although either younger or older patients can be classified into one of 3 distinct groups (based on the relationship between pain, depression, and functional impact), a unique group representing about 25% of older patients also exists.[98] This group is characterized with low pain but high levels of functional impact and fairly high levels of depression.

Other nonpharmacologic therapies, such as interventional approaches, may also need consideration and include treatments such as nerve blocks, nerve ablations, and other nonsurgical and minimally invasive therapies. Although this is another possible avenue for pain management, the evidence base regarding their effectiveness is still not well established for older adults.[99]

## SUMMARY

Pain in older people is a pervasive problem. Overall, the epidemiologic data suggest that the prevalence of musculoskeletal and neuropathic pain increases with age until at least late midlife, although it is still unclear whether these pain types continue to increase beyond that point. It is surprising that musculoskeletal pain may plateau or decline in older adults because the prevalence of radiography-identified musculoskeletal disease continues to increase with age. Although pain prevalence may peak in late midlife, pain is still a substantial and common complaint even in the oldest age groups. Substantial barriers to pain management exist, complicating the treatment of pain among older persons; particularly cognitive impairments and the effect of age on pharmacokinetics. Patient attitudes and health care provider beliefs can be instrumental in the effectiveness of pain treatments. For these reasons, later-life pain management is often complex and nuanced. As described elsewhere in this issue, pain management that adopts a multimodal approach and incorporates both pharmacologic and non-pharmacologic treatment modalities is strongly recommended.

## ACKNOWLEDGMENTS

The authors would like to thank Ms Hannah Capon for technical assistance with the data and figures.

## REFERENCES

1. World Population Prospects - Population Division - United Nations [Internet]. 2015. Available at: http://esa.un.org/unpd/wpp/. Accessed November 25, 2015.
2. Gagliese L. Pain and aging: the emergence of a new subfield of pain research. J Pain 2009;10(4):343–53.
3. Molton IR, Terrill AL. Overview of persistent pain in older adults. Am Psychol 2014;69(2):197–207.
4. Johnson MI, Elzahaf RA, Tashani OA. The prevalence of chronic pain in developing countries. Pain Manag 2013;3(2):83–6.
5. Tsang A, Von Korff M, Lee S, et al. Common chronic pain conditions in developed and developing countries: gender and age differences and comorbidity with depression-anxiety disorders. J Pain 2008;9(10):883–91.
6. Stewart Williams J, Ng N, Peltzer K, et al. Risk factors and disability associated with low back pain in older adults in low- and middle-income countries. Results from the WHO Study on Global AGEing and Adult Health (SAGE). PLoS One 2015;10(6):e0127880.
7. Woolf AD, Pfleger B. Burden of major musculoskeletal conditions. Bull World Health Organ 2003;81(9):646–56.
8. Dowman B, Campbell RM, Zgaga L, et al. Estimating the burden of rheumatoid arthritis in Africa: a systematic analysis. J Glob Health 2012;2(2):020406.
9. Alamanos Y, Voulgari PV, Drosos AA. Incidence and prevalence of rheumatoid arthritis, based on the 1987 American College of Rheumatology Criteria: a systematic review. Semin Arthritis Rheum 2006;36(3):182–8.
10. Abdel-Nasser AM, Rasker JJ, Valkenburg HA. Epidemiological and clinical aspects relating to the variability of rheumatoid arthritis. Semin Arthritis Rheum 1997;27(2):123–40.
11. Bergh I, Steen G, Waern M, et al. Pain and its relation to cognitive function and depressive symptoms: a Swedish population study of 70-year-old men and women. J Pain Symptom Manage 2003;26(4):903–12.
12. Lichtenstein MJ, Dhanda R, Cornell JE, et al. Disaggregating pain and its effect on physical functional limitations. J Gerontol A Biol Sci Med Sci 1998;53(5):M361–71.
13. Blay SL, Andreoli SB, Gastal FL. Chronic painful physical conditions, disturbed sleep and psychiatric morbidity: results from an elderly survey. Ann Clin Psychiatry 2007;19(3):169–74.
14. Blyth FM, March LM, Brnabic AJ, et al. Chronic pain in Australia: a prevalence study. Pain 2001;89(2–3):127–34.
15. Elliott AM, Smith BH, Hannaford PC, et al. The course of chronic pain in the community: results of a 4-year follow-up study. Pain 2002;99(1):299–307.
16. McCarthy LH, Bigal ME, Katz M, et al. Chronic pain and obesity in the elderly: results from the Einstein Aging Study. J Am Geriatr Soc 2009;57(1):115–9.

17. Sá KN, Baptista AF, Matos MA, et al. Chronic pain and gender in Salvador population, Brazil. Pain 2008;139(3):498–506.

18. Yu HY, Tang FI, Kuo BI, et al. Prevalence, interference, and risk factors for chronic pain among Taiwanese community older people. Pain Manag Nurs 2006;7(1):2–11.

19. Elliott AM, Smith BH, Penny KI, et al. The epidemiology of chronic pain in the community. Lancet 1999;354(9186):1248–52.

20. Asghari A, Ghaderi N, Ashory A. The prevalence of pain among residents of nursing homes and the impact of pain on their mood and quality of life. Arch Iran Med 2006;9(4):368–73.

21. Boerlage AA, van Dijk M, Stronks DL, et al. Pain prevalence and characteristics in three Dutch residential homes. Eur J Pain 2008;12(7):910–6.

22. Reis LA, Torres Gde V, Reis LA. Pain characterization in institutionalized elderly patients. Arq Neuropsiquiatr 2008;66(2B):331–5.

23. McClean WJ, Higginbotham NH. Prevalence of pain among nursing home residents in rural New South Wales. Med J Aust 2002;177(1):17–20.

24. Tsai YF, Tsai HH, Lai YH, et al. Pain prevalence, experiences and management strategies among the elderly in Taiwanese nursing homes. J Pain Symptom Manage 2004;28(6):579–84.

25. Weiner D, Peterson B, Ladd K, et al. Pain in nursing home residents: an exploration of prevalence, staff perspectives, and practical aspects of measurement. Clin J Pain 1999;15(2):92–101.

26. Zanocchi M, Maero B, Nicola E, et al. Chronic pain in a sample of nursing home residents: prevalence, characteristics, influence on quality of life (QoL). Arch Gerontol Geriatr 2008;47(1):121–8.

27. Abdulla A, Adams N, Bone M, et al. Guidance on the management of pain in older people. Age Ageing 2013;42(Suppl 1):i1–57.

28. Schmader KE. Epidemiology and impact on quality of life of postherpetic neuralgia and painful diabetic neuropathy. Clin J Pain 2002;18(6):350–4.

29. Bouhassira D, Lantéri-Minet M, Attal N, et al. Prevalence of chronic pain with neuropathic characteristics in the general population. Pain 2008;136(3):380–7.

30. Andersson HI, Ejlertsson G, Leden I, et al. Chronic pain in a geographically defined general population: studies of differences in age, gender, social class, and pain localization. Clin J Pain 1993;9(3):174–82.

31. de Zwart BC, Broersen JP, Frings-Dresen MH, et al. Musculoskeletal complaints in The Netherlands in relation to age, gender and physically demanding work. Int Arch Occup Environ Health 1997;70(5):352–60.

32. Meucci RD, Fassa AG, Faria NM. Prevalence of chronic low back pain: systematic review. Rev Saúde Pública 2015;49.

33. Fejer R, Leboeuf-Yde C. Does back and neck pain become more common as you get older? A systematic literature review. Chiropr Man Therap 2012;20:24.

34. Dionne CE, Dunn KM, Croft PR. Does back pain prevalence really decrease with increasing age? A systematic review. Age Ageing 2006;35(3):229–34.

35. Mehta RH, Rathore SS, Radford MJ, et al. Acute myocardial infarction in the elderly: differences by age. J Am Coll Cardiol 2001;38(3):736–41.

36. Smitherman TA, Burch R, Sheikh H, et al. The prevalence, impact, and treatment of migraine and severe headaches in the United States: a review of statistics from national surveillance studies. Headache 2013;53(3):427–36.

37. Teunissen SC, de Haes HC, Voest EE, et al. Does age matter in palliative care? Crit Rev Oncol Hematol 2006;60(2):152–8.

38. Denard PJ, Holton KF, Miller J, et al. Back pain, neurogenic symptoms, and physical function in relation to spondylolisthesis among elderly men. Spine J 2010;10(10):865–73.
39. Donald IP, Foy C. A longitudinal study of joint pain in older people. Rheumatology 2004;43(10):1256–60.
40. Mailis-Gagnon A, Nicholson K, Yegneswaran B, et al. Pain characteristics of adults 65 years of age and older referred to a tertiary care pain clinic. Pain Res Manag 2008;13(5):389–94.
41. Fejer R, Ruhe A. What is the prevalence of musculoskeletal problems in the elderly population in developed countries? A systematic critical literature review. Chiropr Man Ther 2012;20:31.
42. Patel KV, Guralnik JM, Dansie EJ, et al. Prevalence and impact of pain among older adults in the United States: findings from the 2011 National Health and Aging Trends Study. Pain 2013;154(12):2649–57.
43. Eggermont LH, Bean JF, Guralnik JM, et al. Comparing pain severity versus pain location in the MOBILIZE Boston Study: chronic pain and lower extremity function. J Gerontol A Biol Sci Med Sci 2009;64A(7):763–70.
44. Hartvigsen J, Davidsen M, Hestbaek L, et al. Patterns of musculoskeletal pain in the population: a latent class analysis using a nationally representative interviewer-based survey of 4817 Danes. Eur J Pain 2013;17(3):452–60.
45. Peat DG, Thomas E, Wilkie R, et al. Multiple joint pain and lower extremity disability in middle and old age. Disabil Rehabil 2006;28(24):1543–9.
46. Dunnl KM, Jordan KP, Croft PR. Contributions of prognostic factors for poor outcome in primary care low back pain patients. Eur J Pain 2011;15(3):313–9.
47. Urwin M, Symmons D, Allison T, et al. Estimating the burden of musculoskeletal disorders in the community: the comparative prevalence of symptoms at different anatomical sites, and the relation to social deprivation. Ann Rheum Dis 1998;57(11):649–55.
48. Brochet B, Michel P, Barberger-Gateau P, et al. Population-based study of pain in elderly people: a descriptive survey. Age Ageing 1998;27(3):279–84.
49. Srikanth VK, Fryer JL, Zhai G, et al. A meta-analysis of sex differences prevalence, incidence and severity of osteoarthritis. Osteoarthritis Cartilage 2005;13(9):769–81.
50. Lavin R, Park J. A characterization of pain in racially and ethnically diverse older adults a review of the literature. J Appl Gerontol 2014;33(3):258–90.
51. Hampton SB, Cavalier J, Langford R. The influence of race and gender on pain management: a systematic literature review. Pain Manag Nurs 2015;16(6):968–77.
52. Allison TR, Symmons DP, Brammah T, et al. Musculoskeletal pain is more generalised among people from ethnic minorities than among white people in Greater Manchester. Ann Rheum Dis 2002;61(2):151–6.
53. Choudhury Y, Bremner SA, Ali A, et al. Prevalence and impact of chronic widespread pain in the Bangladeshi and white populations of Tower Hamlets, East London. Clin Rheumatol 2013;32(9):1375–82.
54. Hitt HC, McMillen RC, Thornton-Neaves T, et al. Comorbidity of obesity and pain in a general population: results from the Southern Pain Prevalence Study. J Pain 2007;8(5):430–6.
55. Ray L, Lipton RB, Zimmerman ME, et al. Mechanisms of association between obesity and chronic pain in the elderly. Pain 2011;152(1):53–9.
56. Carroll LJ, Cassidy DJ, Côté P. Depression as a risk factor for onset of an episode of troublesome neck and low back pain. Pain 2004;107(1):134–9.

57. Miaskowski C. The impact of age on a patient's perception of pain and ways it can be managed. Pain Manag Nurs 2000;1(3 Suppl 1):2–7.

58. Cornally N, McCarthy G. Chronic pain: the help-seeking behavior, attitudes, and beliefs of older adults living in the community. Pain Manag Nurs 2011;12(4): 206–17.

59. Yong HH. Can attitudes of stoicism and cautiousness explain observed age-related variation in levels of self-rated pain, mood disturbance and functional interference in chronic pain patients? Eur J Pain 2006;10(5):399.

60. Brown D. A literature review exploring how healthcare professionals contribute to the assessment and control of postoperative pain in older people. J Clin Nurs 2004;13:74–90.

61. Pulvers K, Hood A. The role of positive traits and pain catastrophizing in pain perception. Curr Pain Headache Rep 2013;17(5):330.

62. Darlow B, Fullen BM, Dean S, et al. The association between health care professional attitudes and beliefs and the attitudes and beliefs, clinical management, and outcomes of patients with low back pain: a systematic review. Eur J Pain 2012;16(1):3–17.

63. Husebo BS, Achterberg WP, Lobbezoo F, et al. Pain in patients with dementia: a review of pain assessment and treatment challenges. Nor Epidemiol 2012;22(2): 243–51. Available at: https://www.ntnu.no/ojs/index.php/norepid/article/view/1572.

64. Haasum Y, Fastbom J, Fratiglioni L, et al. Pain treatment in elderly persons with and without dementia: a population-based study of institutionalized and home-dwelling elderly. Drugs Aging 2011;28(4):283–93.

65. Lövheim H, Karlsson S, Gustafson Y. The use of central nervous system drugs and analgesics among very old people with and without dementia. Pharmacoepidemiol Drug Saf 2008;17(9):912–8.

66. Ferrell BA, Ferrell BR, Rivera L. Pain in cognitively impaired nursing home patients. J Pain Symptom Manage 1995;10(8):591–8.

67. Sale JE, Gignac M, Hawker G. How "bad" does the pain have to be? A qualitative study examining adherence to pain medication in older adults with osteoarthritis. Arthritis Rheum 2006;55(2):272–8.

68. Morgan TK, Williamson M, Pirotta M, et al. A national census of medicines use: a 24-hour snapshot of Australians aged 50 years and older. Med J Aust 2012; 196(1):50–3.

69. Dwyer LL, Han B, Woodwell DA, et al. Polypharmacy in nursing home residents in the United States: results of the 2004 National Nursing Home Survey. Am J Geriatr Pharmacother 2010;8(1):63–72.

70. Carragee EJ. Persistent low back pain. N Engl J Med 2005;352(18):1891–8.

71. Jarvik JG, Gold LS, Comstock BA, et al. Association of early imaging for back pain with clinical outcomes in older adults. JAMA 2015;313(11):1143–53.

72. Taylor JA, Bussières A. Diagnostic imaging for spinal disorders in the elderly: a narrative review. Chiropr Man Ther 2012;20:16.

73. Savvas S, Gibson S. Pain management in residential aged care facilities. Aust Fam Physician 2015;44(4):198–203.

74. Bennett M. The LANSS Pain Scale: the Leeds assessment of neuropathic symptoms and signs. Pain 2001;92(1–2):147–57.

75. Backonja MM, Attal N, Baron R, et al. Value of quantitative sensory testing in neurological and pain disorders: NeuPSIG consensus. Pain 2013;154(9): 1807–19.

76. Lawton MP, Brody EM. Assessment of older people: self-maintaining and instrumental activities of daily living. Gerontologist 1969;9(3):179–86.

77. Katz S, Ford AB, Moskowitz RW, et al. Studies of illness in the aged. The index of ADL: a standardized measure of biological and psychosocial function. JAMA 1963;185:914–9.

78. Brink TL, Yesavage JA, Lum O, et al. Screening tests for geriatric depression. Clin Gerontol 1982;1(1):37–43.

79. American Geriatrics Society Panel on Pharmacological Management of Persistent Pain in Older Persons. Pharmacological management of persistent pain in older persons. J Am Geriatr Soc 2009;57(8):1331–46.

80. Pergolizzi J, Böger RH, Budd K, et al. Opioids and the management of chronic severe pain in the elderly: consensus statement of an international expert panel with focus on the six clinically most often used World Health Organization step III opioids (buprenorphine, fentanyl, hydromorphone, methadone, morphine, oxycodone). Pain Pract 2008;8(4):287–313.

81. Makris UE, Abrams RC, Gurland B, et al. Management of persistent pain in the older patient: a clinical review. JAMA 2014;312(8):825–36.

82. Frantsve LM, Kerns RD. Patient-provider interactions in the management of chronic pain: current findings within the context of shared medical decision making. Pain Med 2007;8(1):25–35.

83. Dorflinger L, Kerns RD, Auerbach SM. Providers' roles in enhancing patients' adherence to pain self management. Transl Behav Med 2013;3(1):39–46.

84. Wienecke T, Gøtzsche PC. Paracetamol versus nonsteroidal anti-inflammatory drugs for rheumatoid arthritis. Cochrane Database Syst Rev 2004;(1). CD003789. Available at: http://onlinelibrary.wiley.com.ezp.lib.unimelb.edu.au/doi/10.1002/14651858.CD003789.pub2/abstract.

85. McCarberg BH. NSAIDs in the older patient: balancing benefits and harms. Pain Med 2013;14:S43–4.

86. Franceschi M, Scarcelli C, Niro V, et al. Prevalence, clinical features and avoidability of adverse drug reactions as cause of admission to a geriatric unit: a prospective study of 1756 patients. Drug Saf 2008;31(6):545–56.

87. Chou R, Turner JA, Devine EB, et al. The effectiveness and risks of long-term opioid therapy for chronic pain: a systematic review for a National Institutes of Health Pathways to Prevention workshop. Ann Intern Med 2015;162(4):276–86.

88. Stubbs B, Schofield P, Binnekade T, et al. Pain is associated with recurrent falls in community-dwelling older adults: evidence from a systematic review and meta-analysis. Pain Med 2014;15(7):1115–28.

89. Fishbain DA, Cole B, Lewis J, et al. What percentage of chronic nonmalignant pain patients exposed to chronic opioid analgesic therapy develop abuse/addiction and/or aberrant drug-related behaviors? A structured evidence-based review. Pain Med 2008;9(4):444–59.

90. Noble M, Treadwell JR, Tregear SJ, et al. Long-term opioid management for chronic noncancer pain. Cochrane Database Syst Rev 2010;(1). CD006605. Available at: http://onlinelibrary.wiley.com.ezp.lib.unimelb.edu.au/doi/10.1002/14651858.CD006605.pub2/abstract.

91. Nikolaus T, Zeyfang A. Pharmacological treatments for persistent non-malignant pain in older persons. Drugs Aging 2004;21(1):19–41.

92. Naugle KM, Fillingim RB, Riley JL III. A meta-analytic review of the hypoalgesic effects of exercise. J Pain 2012;13(12):1139–50.

93. Cooney GM, Dwan K, Greig CA, et al. Exercise for depression. Cochrane Database Syst Rev 2013;(9). CD004366. Available at: http://onlinelibrary.wiley.com. ezp.lib.unimelb.edu.au/doi/10.1002/14651858.CD004366.pub6/abstract.

94. Heneweer H, Vanhees L, Picavet HS. Physical activity and low back pain: a U-shaped relation? Pain 2009;143(1–2):21–5.

95. Abenhaim L, Rossignol M, Valat JP, et al. The role of activity in the therapeutic management of back pain. Report of the International Paris Task Force on Back Pain. Spine (Phila Pa 1976) 2000;25(4 Suppl):1S–33S.

96. Gibson SJ, Helme RD. Cognitive factors and the experience of pain and suffering in older persons. Pain 2000;85(3):375–83.

97. Gibson S, Savvas S. Psychological treatment of pain in older populations. In: Gebhart GF, Schmidt RF, editors. Encyclopedia of pain. Berlin: Springer; 2013. p. 3277–83. Available at: http://link.springer.com/referenceworkentry/10. 1007/978-3-642-28753-4_3635.

98. Corran TM, Farrell MJ, Helme RD, et al. The classification of patients with chronic pain: age as a contributing factor. Clin J Pain 1997;13(3):207–14.

99. Chou R, Atlas SJ, Stanos SP, et al. Nonsurgical interventional therapies for low back pain: a review of the evidence for an American pain society clinical practice guideline. Spine 2009;34(10):1078–93.

100. Freburger JK, Holmes GM, Agans RP, et al. The rising prevalence of chronic low back pain. Arch Intern Med 2009;169(3):251–8.

101. Johannes CB, Le TK, Zhou X, et al. The prevalence of chronic pain in United States adults: results of an Internet-based survey. J Pain Off J Am Pain Soc 2010;11(11):1230–9.

102. Silva MC da, Fassa AG, Valle NCJ. Chronic low back pain in a Southern Brazilian adult population: prevalence and associated factors. Cad Saúde Pública 2004; 20(2):377–85.

103. Meucci RD, Fassa AG, Paniz VM, et al. Increase of chronic low back pain prevalence in a medium-sized city of southern Brazil. BMC Musculoskelet Disord 2013;14:155.

104. Andrianakos A, Trontzas P, Christoyannis F, et al. Prevalence of rheumatic diseases in Greece: a cross-sectional population based epidemiological study. The ESORDIG Study. J Rheumatol 2003;30(7):1589–601.

105. Goode AP, Freburger J, Carey T. Prevalence, practice patterns, and evidence for chronic neck pain. Arthritis Care Res 2010;62(11):1594–601.

106. Parsons S, Breen A, Foster NE, et al. Prevalence and comparative troublesomeness by age of musculoskeletal pain in different body locations. Fam Pract 2007;24(4):308–16.

107. Picavet HSJ, Schouten JS. Musculoskeletal pain in the Netherlands: prevalences, consequences and risk groups, the DMC(3)-study. Pain 2003; 102(1–2):167–78.

108. Strine TW, Hootman JM. US national prevalence and correlates of low back and neck pain among adults. Arthritis Rheum 2007;57(4):656–65.

109. Thomas E, Peat G, Harris L, et al. The prevalence of pain and pain interference in a general population of older adults: cross-sectional findings from the North Staffordshire Osteoarthritis Project (NorStOP). Pain 2004;110(1–2):361–8.

# Pain in the Geriatric Patient with Advanced Chronic Disease

Veerawat Phongtankuel, MD[a],*, Prin X. Amorapanth, MD, PhD[b],
Eugenia L. Siegler, MD[a]

## KEYWORDS

- Pain • Geriatric • Congestive heart failure • End-stage renal disease • Stroke
- Opiates

## KEY POINTS

- Although pain is prevalent among patients living with advanced chronic illnesses, it is often overlooked and underreported.
- Pain is commonly intertwined with other physical and psychological symptoms that lead to poorer quality of life.
- End-organ dysfunction influences treatment of pain in patients with advanced chronic illnesses.

## INTRODUCTION

With advances in medical therapies and improvements in public health, individuals are living longer and more productive lives. As a result, more older adults are living with and dying from chronic diseases. More than 85% of Americans 65 years and older have at least one chronic disease. Many suffer from multiple comorbidities, with an estimated 11 million older adults living with 5 or more chronic conditions.[1] Congestive heart failure (CHF), end-stage renal disease (ESRD), and stroke consistently rank among the leading causes of death in the geriatric population.[2]

Many older adults with CHF, ESRD, or stroke experience pain, which can contribute to disability and diminished quality of life. Pain from these diseases is often less well defined and understood than that originating from musculoskeletal (eg, osteoarthritis,

Disclosure Statement: Dr E.L. Siegler receives royalties from Springer Publishing Company. The other authors have nothing to disclose.
[a] Division of Geriatrics and Palliative Medicine, Department of Medicine, Weill Cornell Medical College, 525 East 68th Street Box 39, New York, NY 10065, USA; [b] Department of Rehabilitation, Rusk Rehabilitation at New York University Langone Medical Center, 238 East 38th Street 15-62, New York, NY 10016, USA
* Corresponding author.
E-mail address: vep9012@med.cornell.edu

spinal stenosis) conditions. Furthermore, concerns about medication side effects related to organ dysfunction often complicate the management of pain in these patients. Therefore, this article provides an overview of the epidemiology, etiology, and challenges of treating chronic pain among older adults with CHF, ESRD, or stroke.

## CONGESTIVE HEART FAILURE
### Epidemiology and Prevalence

More than 5 million Americans are living with CHF, and approximately 5% have end-stage disease that is refractory to medical therapies.[3,4] Up to 84% of advanced heart failure patients experience pain, and many report pain in multiple sites.[5] Pain is a significant contributor to the overall symptom burden experienced by patients and can be broadly categorized into 2 types: (1) chronic stable angina and (2) noncardiac pain.

### Etiology of Pain

#### Chronic stable angina
Underlying coronary artery disease is the most common cause of CHF and often leads to chronic stable angina, as inadequate coronary artery perfusion leads to demand-induced myocardial ischemia.[6] Chronic stable angina symptoms are reported in up to 29% of patients with heart disease and classically presents as anterior left-sided chest pain that resolves with rest or nitroglycerin.[7] Stable angina is persistent and chronic over a period of months to years. It is more common for older adults and women to experience atypical presentations of chronic stable angina, which may manifest as dyspnea on exertion, sweats, or lethargy.

#### Noncardiac pain
Although chronic stable angina is a recognized and well-studied entity in cardiology, literature on noncardiac pain in CHF patients is limited. Widely used quality-of-life questionnaires in the CHF population, such as the Minnesota Living with Heart Failure Questionnaire and the Kansas City Cardiomyopathy Questionnaire, do not have questions assessing noncardiac pain.[8,9] However, in one study, 76% of CHF patients report chronic noncardiac pain, which often goes unaddressed by providers.[10] Noncardiac pain in CHF patients is thought to be caused by a combination of complications from refractory disease (ie, skin breakdown from chronic lower extremity edema, peripheral ischemia from poor blood flow), underlying medical comorbidities, and psychosocial stressors.[11,12] Although there are no disease-specific pain assessment tools for patients with heart failure, using the Edmonton Symptom Assessment Scale is a simple standardized way to assess and monitor pain.[13] The Memorial Symptom Assessment Scale can also be used and provides clinicians with a measurement of pain and a multitude of other symptoms.[14]

### Symptoms That Co-occur with Pain

CHF patients often report multiple symptoms. Dyspnea, pain, and low mood are most commonly experienced by patients during their last year of life, whereas loss of appetite, sleeplessness, constipation, nausea, and urinary incontinence contribute to the overall burden of disease.[15] Screening for mood disorders is critical in this population, as 1 in 5 patients meet criteria for major depressive disorder. Depression and pain often co-occur and magnify one another, worsening quality of life.[11] The Patient Health Questionnaire-2 is an effective and quick tool clinicians can use to screen for depression in this patient population.[16]

### Challenges and Management of Pain

As with other chronic diseases, pain in CHF is often under-recognized by doctors and unreported by patients.[17] Although there is good literature on the management of chronic stable angina,[18] there is decidedly less information around noncardiac pain in this patient population, which leaves providers with limited guidance on how to appropriately assess and treat it.

Guidelines in managing noncardiac pain in advanced CHF patients have yet to be established; therefore, providers should use the World Health Organization analgesic ladder as a guide when considering treatment options. The World Health Organization[19] guideline recommends that: (1) analgesics should be administered orally whenever possible, (2) analgesics should be given at regular intervals, (3) analgesics should be prescribed according to pain intensity determined using a validated pain intensity scale, (4) dosing of pain medication should be adapted for each patient because there is no standardized dosage when treating pain, and (5) education should be provided to the patient (and family member or caregiver when appropriate) about the importance of regular administration of analgesic medication. Pain treatment should begin with a nonopioid medication. If pain is not well controlled, a weak opioid should be started. If no relief is achieved with a weak opioid, then a trial of a stronger opioid should be considered. The use of adjuvant medications should be considered in each step of the ladder.

Although guidance on effective treatments is limited, there are established data on certain pharmacologic agents that should be used with caution. Nonsteroidal anti-inflammatory drugs (NSAIDs) are generally avoided given the risk of sodium and fluid retention, which can lead to exacerbation of CHF symptoms. Acetaminophen is recommended for the treatment of mild pain. When prescribing opioids for moderate or severe pain, methadone can prolong the QT interval and requires special attention and periodic electrocardiograms if prescribed.[20] Other opioid medications such as morphine and codeine should be used with caution in CHF patients with renal impairment, as reduced clearance of active renal metabolites can lead to myoclonus, delirium, and other deleterious outcomes. Pregabalin, occasionally used as an adjuvant therapy, is reported to increase edema in CHF patients, and its use should be closely monitored if administered.[12]

Although the evidence regarding nonpharmacologic treatments for pain in the CHF population has been indeterminate, there is evidence that chronic pain is often best treated using a multidisciplinary approach.[21] Therefore, clinicians should consider using cognitive behavioral approaches, physical therapy, and acupuncture as complementary options to treat pain.[22]

## END-STAGE RENAL DISEASE
### Epidemiology and Prevalence

More than 600,000 patients in the United States are living with ESRD, with approximately 100,000 new cases reported in 2012.[23] Symptom burden in this cohort is among the highest when compared with patients living with other chronic diseases. Pain is a significant contributor, with more than 65% of hemodialysis patients experiencing chronic pain.[24]

### Etiology of Pain

#### Chronic kidney disease–mineral and bone disorder
Patients with ESRD on hemodialysis will have some degree of chronic kidney disease–mineral and bone disorder (CKD-MBD), a disorder marked by abnormalities in bone

metabolism, bone turnover, and extraskeletal calcification. The pathologic bone changes attributed to CKD-MBD are termed *renal osteodystrophy* and can lead to bone pain. Adynamic bone disease is the most common type of renal osteodystrophy, in which pain is believed to be a result of poor microdamage repair related to low bone turnover.[25] In addition to bone pain, patients with renal osteodystrophy have a greater than 10-fold risk of fracture, which can lead to significant morbidity and mortality.[26]

### Calciphylaxis

Calciphylaxis is a rare, painful disorder that deserves mention, as it carries significant risk of morbidity and mortality. This condition results from abnormal metabolism of calcium and phosphate, leading to arteriole calcification and painful skin lesions caused by vascular ischemia and necrosis.[27] Patients will experience intense, excruciating pain that is challenging for providers to manage.

### Polycystic kidney disease

Patients with ESRD caused by polycystic kidney disease (PCKD) often experience abdominal, back, and flank pain that is thought to be caused by cyst involvement. Cyst enlargement can stretch the kidney capsule resulting in pain, which is typically dull in nature.[28] Diagnosis can be difficult given that pain can present in various regions of the abdomen and can mimic other gastrointestinal or musculoskeletal conditions. Prevalence of pain occurs in more than 60% of PCKD patients.[29]

### Comorbidities and dialysis-associated pain

Comorbidities and dialysis-associated pain also contribute significantly to the pain experienced by ESRD patients. The most common complaints are musculoskeletal pain, which are often attributed to osteoarthritis. Diabetes, the leading cause of ESRD in the United States, can lead to painful neuropathies and ischemic ulcers.[30] Even the dialysis process itself can result in pain, headaches, and cramping.

### Symptoms That Co-occur with Pain

ESRD patients often experience many other burdensome symptoms that can impair their quality of life.[31] For example, more than 80% of patients report generalized fatigue, which many find to be the most troublesome symptom.[31] In addition, dizziness, headaches, pruritus, constipation, sleep disturbances, restless leg syndrome, anorexia, and nausea are also commonly reported.

Pain is often intertwined with the psychological well-being of patients. ESRD-related pain is associated with excess psychological burden. Anxiety and depression are noted to be as high as 45% and 25% in ESRD patients, respectively.[32,33] The generalized anxiety disorder-7 scale and the Patient Health Questionnaire-2 are simple and important tools that should be used to screen patients in this population.[34]

### Challenges and Management of Pain

A major challenge in managing chronic pain in this population is improving its recognition by clinicians who are often focused on renal replacement therapy. The Edmonton Symptom Assessment Scale and the Palliative Care Outcomes Scale are simple tools that can be implemented to assess pain in these patients.[35,36] Despite the availability of these tools, under-recognition of pain in ESRD patients is common,[37] and even moderate-to-severe chronic pain may go untreated.[38] Even when pain is recognized and managed, patients may be inadequately treated. Approximately 38% of ESRD patients taking opioids still report moderate-to-severe pain.[30] Reasons behind undertreatment and underdosing of analgesic medications are multifactorial and include providers' concerns of the adverse side effects of analgesic use in ESRD, inadequate assessment of pain, and patients' reluctance to use more potent analgesics.

### Chronic kidney disease–mineral and bone disorder, calciphylaxis, polycystic kidney disease

Treatment for CKD-MBD currently involves determining and treating the underlying metabolic disorders, most of which have parathyroid abnormalities as the underlying cause.[25] Treatment focuses on reducing risk factors, which consists of avoiding calcium-based phosphate binders, active vitamin D analogs, and high-dialysate calcium concentration. Calciphylaxis is a challenging disorder to manage. Treatment consists of a multidisciplinary approach that can include wound care, opioids, and oxygen therapy.[27] Pain management for PCKD includes pharmacologic drugs such as acetaminophen, tramadol, and clonidine. Patients who are refractory to pharmacologic treatments can be referred for laparoscopic cyst decortication and nerve denervation.[28]

### Other treatments

The presence of ESRD introduces distinct challenges that providers must be aware of when deciding on appropriate analgesic medication and dosing. In ESRD patients with mild-to-moderate pain, acetaminophen and NSAIDs are commonly used. Acetaminophen is preferred, as it is metabolized in the liver, does not require dose adjustments, and does not influence platelet function. NSAIDs, if used, should be administered for short periods and for specific indications (eg, gout flares). Although NSAIDS have greater anti-inflammatory properties than acetaminophen (and concerns about effects on kidney function are no longer relevant), providers must keep in mind their effect on platelet function and gastric mucosa, which may lead to increased risk of bleeding.[39] The use of selective cyclooxygenase-2 (COX-2) inhibitors may reduce the risk of gastritis; however, these selective COX-2 inhibitors and nonselective NSAIDs can elevate blood pressure and lead to increased risk of heart attacks and strokes.[40]

Opioids are generally needed for adequate relief of moderate-to-severe pain. Tramadol has been used to treat pain in ESRD patients; however, it is mainly cleared by the kidneys and its dose needs to be renally adjusted. Clinicians should also assess a patient's risk for seizure before prescribing a trial. Although there are limited data on the use of oxycodone and hydromorphone, they are commonly prescribed because they are cheap and have short half-lives.[41] Morphine and codeine are not recommended for ESRD patients and should be avoided. Codeine can cause respiratory depression, hypotension, and narcolepsy.[42] Morphine is not recommended in this population, as its active metabolites, which are renally excreted, can accumulate, resulting in myoclonus, seizures, and respiratory depression. More potent opioids such as fentanyl and methadone are recommended for use for severe pain, as there is no accumulation of active metabolites.

The literature on nonpharmacologic treatments for pain in ESRD patients is limited. However, treatments such as cognitive behavioral therapies, physical therapy, and yoga should be tried in conjunction with pharmacologic treatment when available and if beneficial to the patient.[43]

## STROKE
### Epidemiology and Prevalence

Stroke affects almost 800,000 people annually in the United States and is a leading cause of long-term disability.[44] In addition to well-recognized impairments in motor function, cognition, and language, stroke can also result in pain that is difficult to diagnosis and treat.

Poststroke pain (PSP) affects more than half of all stroke patients and results in decreased function and quality of life.[45] Pain may be broadly categorized as either neurologic or musculoskeletal in origin. Because of differences in definition and identification, the reported prevalence of PSP varies, ranging from 4% to 66%.[46,47] Common types of PSP encountered include central poststroke pain (CPSP), muscle spasticity, and poststroke shoulder pain.[47,48]

## Etiology of Pain

### Central poststroke pain

CPSP is a type of central neuropathic pain typically characterized by dysesthestic and allodynic qualities on the side contralateral to the stroke.[49] Although CPSP affects up to one-third of stroke patients, its insidious onset and subacute natural history complicate diagnosis, as CPSP usually does not present until at least a month after stroke onset.[50,51] Most cases present within a year.[52] The pain of CPSP can be especially severe and intractable, posing a significant therapeutic challenge.[51]

### Muscle spasticity

Muscle spasticity–related pain is another common source of chronic pain experienced by stroke patients and develops in nearly 25% of patients within 1 week of stroke.[53] Most stroke patients with spasticity will go on to have pain in the affected limb(s).[53] Although a clear mechanism by which spasticity results in pain has not been identified, it is hypothesized that abnormal tensile load on muscles and ligaments leads to nociceptive pain.[54]

### Poststroke shoulder pain

Poststroke shoulder pain is a common cause of pain after stroke, affecting up to 72% of stroke patients[55,56] and occurring soon after stroke (within 3 weeks).[55] The etiology of shoulder pain is multifactorial and may include mechanical factors such as glenohumeral joint subluxation or impingement, rotator cuff tears, and bicipital tendonitis.

## Symptoms That Co-occur with Pain

As with pain more generally, PSP interacts broadly within the brain and is influenced by multiple factors such as mood, sleep, stress, and general health. Along with the potential cognitive and functional deficits caused by stroke, poststroke patients often experience fatigue, depression, and poorer quality of life. PSP has been found to be a predictor of suicidality after stroke.[45,46,48,54] Within the various types of PSP, other symptoms and findings may cluster. Emotional stimuli, such as negative emotions like fear, sadness, or anger, may elicit or exacerbate pain.

## Challenges and Management of Pain

PSP is characterized by multiple patient-centered and systemic challenges related to its evaluation and management. Diagnostic challenges include patients who are unable to provide an accurate history of their pain because of cognitive deficits and those who may be reluctant to volunteer pain-related symptoms. Quantification of PSP is particularly complicated by the lack of a PSP-specific rating scale. Commonly encountered scales may be numeric, visual, or verbal, and use of a particular tool needs to be tailored to the impairments of a given patient. Utilization of visual scales or locative diagrams, such as the Wong-Baker FACES Pain Rating Scale or the McGill Pain Questionnaire, may be more useful than a verbal or numeric rating scale.[57,58]

In addition, PSP patients often have multiple medical comorbidities that frequently complicate both the diagnosis and management of pain. Polypharmacy and adverse side effects of analgesic medications in this population can threaten cognition and arousal and limit pharmacologic treatment options.

Management of PSP typically involves a focus on both central and peripheral targets. Depending on the subtype of PSP, interventions aim to address peripheral inflammation, relay of nociceptive input at the spinal cord, central maladaptive neuroplasticity, or mood impairments. Although several classes of medications have shown efficacy in treating PSP, many of these medications have adverse side effects on mental status and cognition. Therefore, it is crucial to regularly assess whether the medication is still necessary for pain control and is continuing to provide benefit to the patient.

For CPSP, pharmacologic therapies fall broadly into several categories: aminergic agents, calcium channel blockers, GABAergic agents, glutamate antagonists, and membrane stabilizers. Amitriptyline and lamotrigine are considered first-line treatments for CPSP, although adverse anticholinergic side effects frequently limit use.[59] Mexiletine, fluvoxamine, and gabapentin have been used as second-line drugs. Patients who are refractory to pharmacotherapy may benefit from referral to pain management specialists for neuromodulatory interventions, which include transcranial or deep brain stimulatory technologies.

Treatment options for spasticity run the spectrum from nonpharmacologic strategies to pharmacologic and interventional approaches.[60] Stretching, splinting, and strengthening of antagonist muscles by trained physical and occupational therapists form an important cornerstone of spasticity treatment. Oral medications, such as baclofen, tizanidine, diazepam, and dantrolene, may facilitate the effect of stretching and other therapies. Because sedation is a common side effect for many of these medications, generally accepted practice is to start at the lowest dose before bed and then titrating up in dose and frequency. For focal spasticity, focal injections of phenol or botulinum toxin have shown efficacy in reducing tone and improving function.

In the immediate poststroke period, the combination of muscle flaccidity and joint laxity combine to produce a window of increased vulnerability to injury. Thus, a preventive approach to joint injury in conjunction with early physical/occupational therapy, as well as appropriate mechanical support and mobility control, may reduce the incidence of poststroke shoulder pain.[61] Medications used for poststroke shoulder pain center around the control of inflammation, with NSAIDs often used first.[61] Topical analgesic medications in the form of creams (ie, lidocaine, capsaicin), gels (ie, diclofenac, ketoprofen, ibuprofen), or patches (ie, lidocaine, diclofenac) may be used to provide targeted pain relief. To the degree that muscle spasticity contributes to pain, antispasmodic agents such as baclofen may also be useful. Transcutaneous neuromuscular electrical stimulation and functional electrical stimulation may also be used to improve pain, range of motion, and arm function.[62] If focal pathology at one of the many joints comprising the shoulder is suspected, targeted delivery of combined anesthetic and corticosteroid may be used for both immediate pain relief and longer-term inflammatory control. For refractory cases of shoulder pain in which permanent mechanical contracture or defect is suspected, surgery may represent definitive treatment to release contracted shoulder muscles or rotator cuff tears.

## SUMMARY

Pain is a common and debilitating symptom experienced by many patients with advanced chronic disease. In patients with CHF, ESRD, and stroke, pain is often underassessed and undertreated. Therefore, providers need to be proactive in implementing routine and standardized ways to evaluate pain in these patients. Furthermore, it is important that providers understand what treatment options are appropriate for use in the setting of advanced organ dysfunction. Ultimately, therapies should be tailored to align with the goals of the patient, whether it is palliative or functional in intent. Although pharmacologic therapies are a mainstay in treating pain, pain is often interwoven with other physical and psychological symptoms. Therefore, a multidisciplinary and multipronged approach is key when managing pain in patients living with advanced chronic disease.

## ACKNOWLEDGMENTS

The authors acknowledge the significant contribution of Shawn Paustian who assisted in the literature review and writing of the article.

## REFERENCES

1. AARP. Chronic Conditions among older Americans. Available at: http://assets. aarp.org/rgcenter/health/beyond_50_hcr_conditions.pdf. Accessed November 11, 2015.
2. CDC. 10 leading causes of death by age group, United States - 2013. 2013. Available at: http://www.cdc.gov/injury/images/lc-charts/leading_causes_of_death_by_age_group_2013-a.gif. Accessed December 2, 2015.
3. Adler ED, Goldfinger JZ, Kalman J, et al. Palliative care in the treatment of advanced heart failure. Circulation 2009;120(25):2597–606.
4. Go AS, Mozaffarian D, Roger VL, et al. Heart disease and stroke statistics–2013 update: a report from the American Heart Association. Circulation 2013;127(1): e6–245.
5. Goodlin SJ, Wingate S, Albert NM, et al. Investigating pain in heart failure patients: the pain assessment, incidence, and nature in heart failure (PAIN-HF) study. J Card Fail 2012;18(10):776–83.
6. Abrams J. Chronic stable angina. N Engl J Med 2005;352:2524–33.
7. Beltrame JF, Weekes AJ, Morgan C, et al. The prevalence of weekly angina among patients with chronic stable angina in primary care practices: the Coronary Artery Disease in General Practice (CADENCE) Study. Arch Intern Med 2009;169(16):1491–9.
8. Green CP, Porter CB, Bresnahan DR, et al. Development and evaluation of the Kansas City Cardiomyopathy Questionnaire: a new health status measure for heart failure. J Am Coll Cardiol 2000;35(5):1245–55.
9. Rector TS, Cohn JN. Assessment of patient outcome with the Minnesota Living with Heart Failure questionnaire: reliability and validity during a randomized, double-blind, placebo-controlled trial of pimobendan. Pimobendan Multicenter Research Group. Am Heart J 1992;124(4):1017–25.
10. McDonald DD, Soutar C, Chan MA, et al. A closer look: alternative pain management practices by heart failure patients with chronic pain. Heart Lung 2015;44(5): 395–9.
11. Lemond L, Allen LA. Palliative care and hospice in advanced heart failure. Prog Cardiovasc Dis 2011;54(2):168–78.
12. DeJongh B, Birkeland K, Brenner M. Managing comorbidities in patients with chronic heart failure: first, do no harm. Am J Cardiovasc Drugs 2015;15(3): 171–84.

13. Bruera E, Kuehn N, Miller MJ, et al. The Edmonton Symptom Assessment System (ESAS): a simple method for the assessment of palliative care patients. J Palliat Care 1991;7(2):6–9.

14. Portenoy RK, Thaler HT, Kornblith AB, et al. The Memorial Symptom Assessment Scale: an instrument for the evaluation of symptom prevalence, characteristics and distress. Eur J Cancer 1994;30A(9):1326–36.

15. Nordgren L, Sorensen S. Symptoms experienced in the last six months of life in patients with end-stage heart failure. Eur J Cardiovasc Nurs 2003;2:213–7.

16. Kroenke K, Spitzer RL, Williams JBW. The Patient Health Questionnaire-2: validity of a two-item depression screener. Med Care 2003;41(11):1284–92.

17. Conley S, Feder S, Redeker NS. The relationship between pain, fatigue, depression and functional performance in stable heart failure. Heart Lung 2015;44(2):107–12.

18. Fihn SD, Gardin JM, Abrams J, et al. 2012 ACCF/AHA/ACP/AATS/PCNA/SCAI/STS guideline for the diagnosis and management of patients with stable ischemic heart disease: a report of the American College of Cardiology Foundation/American Heart Association Task Force on Practice Guidelines, and the. Circulation 2012;126(25):e354–471.

19. World Health Organization. Traitement de la douleur cancéreuse. Geneva, Switzerland: World Health Organization; 1997.

20. Light-McGroary K, Goodlin SJ. The challenges of understanding and managing pain in the heart failure patient. Curr Opin Support Palliat Care 2013;7(1):14–20.

21. Scascighini L, Toma V, Dober-Spielmann S, et al. Multidisciplinary treatment for chronic pain: a systematic review of interventions and outcomes. Rheumatology (Oxford) 2008;47(5):670–8.

22. Kwekkeboom KL, Bratzke LC. A systematic review of relaxation, meditation, and guided imagery strategies for symptom management in heart failure. J Cardiovasc Nurs 2015. [Epub ahead of print].

23. System USRD. 2012 USRDS Annual Data Report. 2012. Available at: http://www.usrds.org/2012/view/v2_01.aspx. Accessed November 21, 2015.

24. Almutary H, Bonner A, Douglas C. Symptom burden in chronic kidney disease: a review of recent literature. J Ren Care 2013;39(3):140–50, 5498.

25. Moe S, Drüeke T, Cunningham J, et al. Definition, evaluation, and classification of renal osteodystrophy: a position statement from Kidney Disease: improving Global Outcomes (KDIGO). Kidney Int 2006;69(11):1945–53.

26. Coco M, Rush H. Increased incidence of hip fractures in dialysis patients with low serum parathyroid hormone. Am J Kidney Dis 2000;36(6):1115–21.

27. Nigwekar SU, Kroshinsky D, Nazarian RM, et al. Calciphylaxis: risk factors, diagnosis, and treatment. Am J Kidney Dis 2015;66(1):133–46.

28. Tellman MW, Bahler CD, Shumate AM, et al. Management of pain in autosomal dominant polycystic kidney disease and anatomy of renal innervation. J Urol 2015;193(5):1470–8.

29. Gabow PA. Autosomal dominant polycystic kidney disease. N Engl J Med 1993;329(5):332–42.

30. Davison SN. Pain in hemodialysis patients: prevalence, cause, severity, and management. Am J Kidney Dis 2003;42(6):1239–47.

31. Almantary H. Symptom burden in chronic kidney disease: a review of recent literature. J Clin Nurs 2014;23(13–14):2031–42.

32. Cukor D, Ver Halen N, Fruchter Y. Anxiety and quality of life in ESRD. Semin Dial 2013;26(3):265–8.

33. Palmer S, Vecchio M, Craig JC, et al. Prevalence of depression in chronic kidney disease: systematic review and meta-analysis of observational studies. Kidney Int 2013;84(1):179–91.

34. Robert L, Spitzer M, Kurt Kroenke M, et al. A brief measure for assessing generalized anxiety disorder the GAD-7. Arch Intern Med 2006;166(10):1092–7.

35. Murphy EL, Murtagh FEM, Carey I, et al. Understanding symptoms in patients with advanced chronic kidney disease managed without dialysis: use of a short patient-completed assessment tool. Nephron Clin Pract 2009;111(1):c74–80.

36. Hearn J, Higginson IJ. Development and validation of a core outcome measure for palliative care: the palliative care outcome scale. Qual Health Care 1999; 8(4):219–27.

37. Upadhyay C, Cameron K, Murphy L, et al. Measuring pain in patients undergoing hemodialysis: a review of pain assessment tools. Clin Kidney J 2014;7(4):367–72.

38. Davison SN. The prevalence and management of chronic pain in end-stage renal disease. J Palliat Med 2007;10(6):1277–87.

39. Kurella M, Bennett WM, Chertow GM. Analgesia in patients with ESRD: a review of available evidence. Am J Kidney Dis 2003;42(2):217–28.

40. FDA Drug Safety Communication: FDA strengthens warning that non-aspirin nonsteroidal anti-inflammatory drugs (NSAIDs) can cause heart attacks or strokes. 2015. Available at: http://www.fda.gov/Drugs/DrugSafety/ucm451800. htm. Accessed November 28, 2015.

41. Murtagh FEM, Chai MO, Donohoe P, et al. The use of opioid analgesia in end-stage renal disease patients managed without dialysis. J Pain Palliat Care Pharmacother 2007;21(2):5–16.

42. O'Connor NR, Corcoran AM. End-stage renal disease: symptom management and advance care planning. Am Fam Physician 2012;85:705–10.

43. Yurtkuran M, Alp A, Dilek K. A modified yoga-based exercise program in hemodialysis patients: a randomized controlled study. Complement Ther Med 2007; 15(3):164–71.

44. Mozaffarian D, Benjamin EJ, Go AS, et al. Heart disease and stroke statistics-2015 update: a report from the American Heart Association. Circulation 2014; 131(4):e29–322.

45. Naess H, Lunde L, Brogger J. The effects of fatigue, pain, and depression on quality of life in ischemic stroke patients: the Bergen Stroke Study. Vasc Health Risk Manag 2012;8:407–13.

46. Jönsson A-C, Lindgren I, Hallström B, et al. Prevalence and intensity of pain after stroke: a population based study focusing on patients' perspectives. J Neurol Neurosurg Psychiatry 2006;77(5):590–5.

47. Hansen AP, Marcussen NS, Klit H, et al. Pain following stroke: a prospective study. Eur J Pain 2012;16(8):1128–36.

48. O'Donnell MJ, Diener H-C, Sacco RL, et al. Chronic pain syndromes after ischemic stroke: PRoFESS trial. Stroke 2013;44(5):1238–43.

49. Nasreddine ZS, Saver JL. Pain after thalamic stroke: right diencephalic predominance and clinical features in 180 patients. Neurology 1997;48(5):1196–9.

50. Widar M, Samuelsson L, Karlsson-Tivenius S, et al. Long-term pain conditions after a stroke. J Rehabil Med 2002;34(4):165–70.

51. Leijon G, Boivie J, Johansson I. Central post-stroke pain — neurological symptoms and pain characteristics. Pain 1989;36(1):13–25.

52. Canavero S, Bonicalzi V. Central pain of brain origin: epidemiology and clinical features. New York: Cambridge University Press; 1989.

53. Wissel J, Schelosky LD, Scott J, et al. Early development of spasticity following stroke: a prospective, observational trial. J Neurol 2010;257(7):1067–72.
54. Lundström E, Smits A, Terént A, et al. Risk factors for stroke-related pain 1 year after first-ever stroke. Eur J Neurol 2009;16(2):188–93.
55. Dromerick AW, Edwards DF, Kumar A. Hemiplegic shoulder pain syndrome: frequency and characteristics during inpatient stroke rehabilitation. Arch Phys Med Rehabil 2008;89(8):1589–93.
56. Lindgren I, Jönsson A-C, Norrving B, et al. Shoulder pain after stroke: a prospective population-based study. Stroke 2007;38(2):343–8.
57. Wong DL, Hockenberry-Eaton M, Wilson D. Wong's essentials of pediatric nursing. 6th edition. St. Louis (MO): Mosby; 2001.
58. Melzack R. The McGill Pain Questionnaire: Major properties and scoring methods. Pain 1975;1(3):277–99.
59. Kumar B, Kalita J, Kumar G, et al. Central poststroke pain: a review of pathophysiology and treatment. Anesth Analg 2009;108(5):1645–57.
60. Marciniak C. Poststroke hypertonicity: upper limb assessment and treatment. Top Stroke Rehabil 2011;18(3):179–94.
61. Dawson AS, Knox J, McClure JA, et al. Stroke Best Practice Working Group Stroke rehabilitation; 2013. Available at: http://strokebestpractices.ca/wp-content/uploads/2013/07/SBP2013_Stroke-Rehabilitation-Update_July-10_FINAL.pdf. Accessed December 1, 2015.
62. Faghri PD, Rodgers MM, Glaser RM, et al. The effects of functional electrical stimulation on shoulder subluxation, arm function recovery, and shoulder pain in hemiplegic stroke patients. Arch Phys Med Rehabil 1994;75(1):73–9.

# Impact of Pain on Family Members and Caregivers of Geriatric Patients

Catherine Riffin, PhD[a],*, Terri Fried, MD[a,b], Karl Pillemer, PhD[c]

## KEYWORDS

- Geriatric pain • Family members • Spouses • Interpersonal relationships
- Relationship closeness • Coping • Pain perception

## KEY POINTS

- Persistent pain contributes to relationship problems, psychological distress, and physical morbidity among patients and their family members.
- Theory and research implicate several mechanisms that may moderate the effects of older adults' pain on their family members: relationship closeness, coping behavior, pain perception, and communication.
- Most studies investigating the interpersonal consequences of pain combine middle-aged (<64) and older adults (>65) into a single sample; limited research has explicitly examined the effects of pain among older persons (>65) on family members.
- Most research investigating the impact of geriatric pain on family members comes from spousal samples; little is known about the consequences for adult children.
- Future studies should conduct subgroup analyses by age and comparisons of family member outcomes by relationship (spouses vs adult children) and caregiver status.

The interpersonal consequences of chronic pain have been vigorously examined in adolescent, young adult, and middle-aged samples. A wide body of research suggests that persistent pain in the early years of life not only afflicts the individual sufferer, but also close family members involved in his or her care.[1–4] In view of this evidence, consensus statements[5] and clinical guidelines[6] have emphasized the

Disclosure Statement: C. Riffin is supported by a National Institute on Aging Training Grant (T32AG1934).
<sup>a</sup> Department of Internal Medicine, Yale School of Medicine, 333 Cedar Street, New Haven, CT 06520, USA; <sup>b</sup> Clinical Epidemiology Unit, Geriatrics and Extended Care, Department of Internal Medicine (Geriatrics), Veterans Affairs Connecticut Healthcare System, 950 Campbell Avenue, West Haven, CT 06516, USA; <sup>c</sup> Department of Human Development, College of Human Ecology, Cornell University, MVR G77, Ithaca, NY 06902, USA
* Corresponding author. Department of Medicine (Geriatrics), Yale School of Medicine, 333 Cedar Street, PO Box 208239, New Haven, CT 06520.
E-mail address: catherine.riffin@yale.edu

need to address family considerations as part of standard care. However, although the negative effects of pain have been well established among the family members of young persons, a small but growing body of research has begun to examine this phenomenon among the relatives of older persons. Studies in this area are slowly emerging as clinicians, researchers, and policy makers acknowledge the increasing prevalence of pain among older people[7–9] and escalating demand for informal caregiving by relatives.[10]

The interpersonal effects of chronic pain may differ in later life, given pronounced age differences in individuals' physical disability,[11] overall perception of the pain experience,[12] and because chronic pain is often one of many burdensome health conditions that older adults and their family members must confront.[13] As such, specific attention to the effects of pain on family members and caregivers of older persons is warranted.

This article provides an overview of the growing, yet limited, literature on the effects of geriatric patients' pain on their family members. The review focuses on three key consequences for family members: (1) deterioration in relationship functioning, (2) diminished emotional well-being, and (3) compromised physical health. For each consequence, we identify the relevant theoretic frameworks that explain the relationship between geriatric patients' pain and family member's outcomes, highlight the mechanisms that may moderate the effects of patients' pain on family members' well-being and relationships, and present the available empirical evidence of these associations. Given the paucity of research examining the effects of geriatric patients' pain on their relatives, we conclude with several recommendations for future research and clinical practice.

## OLDER ADULT'S PAIN AND RELATIONSHIP FUNCTIONING

When considering the interpersonal consequences of pain, researchers point to the reciprocal interactions between the patient with chronic pain and family members. Just as family members play an important role in the patient's adjustment to and recovery from illness, they are also affected by the patient's symptoms and need for assistance. For middle-aged and older adults, severe pain contributes to increased interpersonal conflict and discord,[14–21] and decreased emotional closeness and physical intimacy.[22–25]

The family systems perspective has been influential in explicating such effects. According to this framework, family functioning is governed by specific social norms and principles.[26,27] When a relative is in pain, family members adjust their social roles to accommodate the sufferer's physical, social, and recreational restrictions. Consequently, these adjustments may lead to a paradoxic cycle of accentuated closeness and enmeshment, followed by tension and strain within the relationship, and ultimately withdrawal by the patient.[28,29] For example, qualitative research has shown that worsening pain symptoms may impact the pain sufferer's ability to maintain employment or complete household activities,[20] thereby leading him or her to become dependent on relatives. In response, family members who take on these tasks experience resentment and hostility toward the patient, along with feelings of guilt and self-blame and a sense of helplessness about how best to provide effective support for their loved one.[20,22,23] Over time, family members may resort to controlling or soliciting behavior, further contributing to patients' distancing from the relationship, and perpetuating the cycle of extreme closeness and withdrawal.[20,23]

However, not all families follow this downward trajectory. Research has begun to uncover how specific moderators, including pain perception, coping behavior, and pain communication, distinguish families who suffer from poor relationship quality from those who maintain healthy, satisfied relationships. Insights from these studies offer additional information about the interpersonal nature of chronic pain.

## Pain Perception

Both theory and research suggest that family members are often poor judges of patients' pain.[28,30] Studies have shown that spouses may either overestimate[31] or underestimate family members' pain,[32] both of which may have consequences for the interpersonal exchanges within the dyad. Whereas overestimation of pain can lead to reinforcement of the patients' sick role and overprotection by spouses,[31] underestimation may lead to greater criticism and less support by the family member.[33] Importantly, accurate pain perception may facilitate appropriate care provision and supportive responses by spouses. For example, recent research has shown that spouses of older patients with osteoarthritis (OA) who were more accurate judges of their partners' pain offered emotional support that was more satisfying to patients, and also reported less caregiving stress.[30] Although studies have yet to examine the direct association between pain perception and relationship quality or satisfaction, this may be an intriguing hypothesis for future investigation.

## Coping Behavior

Several theories point to coping as an important component in determining relational outcomes among families with a member in pain.[26,34] Cognitive-behavioral models propose that patients' and family members' behaviors and attitudes about the pain experience will inform their interpersonal exchanges and interactions. For example, the Communal Coping Hypothesis[35,36] posits that some patients with chronic pain use catastrophizing (an intensified emotional reaction to the pain experience) to gain intimacy and closeness with others, and to solicit instrumental support. Although researchers have speculated that patient catastrophizing is associated with greater interpersonal problems,[37] no research has explicitly examined this hypothesis among geriatric pain patients and their relatives. Furthermore, related work conducted on middle-aged and older adults failed to detect a relationship between patients' somatizing and marital adjustment (ie, accommodation of a husband and wife to each other).[38] Therefore, additional research is needed to explore the specific effects of older patients' catastrophizing on their family members.

A separate model of coping, the Transactional Model of Health, integrates concepts from family systems and cognitive behavioral theories.[39,40] Although originally developed for families of patients suffering from general medical conditions, it has since been applied within the pain context. According to this framework, the family develops a relatively stable set of beliefs about illness, pain, disability, and coping. These beliefs are proposed to influence the family's appraisal of pain experiences and response to emerging challenges. Interventions drawing on this framework have developed dyadic coping skills training for middle-aged and older patients with OA and their spouses. Such programs have reported greater marital satisfaction among patients with chronic pain, but not among spouses.[41,42] A cross-sectional study of middle-aged and older patients with OA suggests that individuals who engage in more passive coping strategies (ie, escape into fantasy) experience lower marital satisfaction.[43] Given that prior studies simultaneously assess the outcomes of middle-aged and older adults, it is important for future work to examine coping strategies specifically among older adults and their relatives, and to examine differences by age (middle aged vs older adults).

### Pain Communication

A third mechanism that is proposed to moderate the association between geriatric pain and relationship functioning is pain communication, including verbal pain disclosure[44] and nonverbal behavior (eg, displays of physical suffering).[45,46] According to the Operant Conditioning Model of Chronic Pain, verbal and nonverbal forms of communication are used to convey patients' desire for support, attention, and intimacy,[47,48] and to elicit empathic responses from others.[32,49] In turn, affected patients' communication may be maintained by social reinforcement (eg, the sympathetic response of significant others).

Early research examining the effects of nonverbal behaviors on marital satisfaction among patients with low back pain found that the use of nonverbal behaviors was associated with lower marital satisfaction among female, but not male spouses.[27] The authors hypothesize that this effect may be a result of women's skill at recognizing nonverbal cues of pain and distress.[50–52] However, more recent research focusing on verbal communication failed to detect significant associations between the frequency of verbal disclosure among middle-aged patients with chronic pain and spouses' marital satisfaction,[53] although men and women were not considered separately. These somewhat mixed findings point to the need for further examination of verbal and nonverbal communication, their direct associations with marital satisfaction, and potential differences by gender and pain condition.

## IMPACT OF PAIN ON FAMILY MEMBERS' PSYCHOLOGICAL WELL-BEING

In addition to poor relationship functioning, relatives of geriatric pain sufferers are also at increased risk of experiencing diminished psychological well-being and elevated stress. The direct effect of individuals' pain severity on spouses' anxiety and depressive symptoms has been documented in cross-sectional[25,54] and longitudinal research,[55] with qualitative research exposing extreme distress and psychological burden among spouses of middle-aged and older patients with rheumatoid arthritis who suffer from pain.[19] There is also evidence that family members' negative emotions mirror patients' own emotional distress about their symptoms.[54] Studies have shown high levels of congruence in anger and depression among older dyads coping with OA.[56]

Efforts have also been made to identify the specific factors that may place family members at greater risk of negative psychological consequences. In particular, research has considered how such effects may be moderated by relationship closeness and pain communication (discussed next).

### Relationship Closeness

Theoretic models posit that family members' psychological reactions to individuals suffering from chronic pain may vary by the closeness of their relationship.[57] It is suggested that family members who report greater levels of closeness may feel more emotionally connected to their loved one, and therefore share their partner's experience of suffering more intensely. This hypothesis has been supported by longitudinal research with older patients with OA and their spouses. Among dyads reporting greater closeness, increased pain severity in patients was associated with increases in depressive symptoms and decreases in positive affect in spouses over a 6-month period,[58] a finding that held while controlling for baseline levels of illness severity and well-being among spouses and patients. Such results suggest that relationship closeness may play a role in predicting which older couples are at greater risk of negative psychological effects of partners' pain suffering. However, additional research is needed to confirm this association, given that this was the single study to examine such effects.

## Pain Communication

The effects of patients' pain on family members' emotional well-being may also be influenced by the extent to which a patient engages in verbal or nonverbal communication about his or her symptoms.[23] Longitudinal research, for example, has shown that verbal expressions of pain may exacerbate the association between an older individual's level of pain and their spouses' depressive symptoms. In a recent study, husbands whose wives reported severe OA pain and who engaged in high degrees of pain expression (verbal disclosure and nonverbal behavior) experienced significant increases in depressive symptoms over a 6-month period; whereas husbands whose wives reported similarly high levels of pain, but disclosed less, did not show such increases.[55] Similar results have been demonstrated in cross-sectional research with older patients with OA, where wives' pain behavior (rubbing joints and limping) exacerbated husbands' depressive symptoms and anger.[56] Although these studies point to a potential pathway by which pain communication may impact family member's psychological health, future research should aim to replicate these effects.

### Self-efficacy in pain communication

Researchers have hypothesized that self-efficacy in communication may further distinguish patients' and spouses' emotional reactions to the pain experience. For patients, it is thought that low self-efficacy in pain communication may compromise their ability to appropriately discuss pain-related concerns and solicit helpful responses by their loved ones.[59] For spouses, it is suggested that low self-efficacy may elicit negative affective responses, such as worry and frustration.[59] However, only one study has explored these potential associations. Using self-report data from middle-aged and older patients with OA and their partners, the study examined whether self-efficacy in pain communication was associated with positive and negative affect in both members of the dyad. The study's findings were generally consistent with the hypothesized pattern of effects: spouses with high levels of self-efficacy had higher positive affect, and spouses of patients with high self-efficacy were less likely to report negative affect.[59] Although this study provides useful insights into the role of self-efficacy of pain communication in affective responses, replication of these findings is needed before strong conclusions can be made.

## IMPACT OF PAIN ON PHYSICAL FUNCTIONING

Although no studies have explored the effects of geriatric patients' pain on family members physical functioning, emerging evidence points to several negative health consequences for middle-aged spouses, including increased blood pressure, sleep disturbance, and gastrointestinal distress.[60] Research has shown that compared with spouses of healthy adults, middle-aged spouses of patients with chronic pain experience poorer well-being and report experiencing a greater number of chronic conditions (eg, diabetes, heart disease, and high blood pressure)[60,61]; they are also more likely to report a diagnosis of chronic pain themselves.[23]

## Relationship Closeness

Recent evidence suggests that patients' pain may affect spouses' abilities to engage in restorative health behaviors (ie, sleep), and that this association may further depend on closeness of the relationship. Specifically, research has shown adverse associations between older patients' pain and spouses' sleep quality, with the strongest impact on couples who reported high levels of closeness.[62] Given the dearth of literature on this topic, future work is needed to examine the associations between patients' pain, spouses' health behaviors, and physical well-being.

## FUTURE DIRECTIONS

Although the existing literature on geriatric patient pain remains sparse, the available evidence demonstrates important links between chronic pain experienced by older adults and family members' outcomes. The previous studies reviewed indicate that persistent pain among geriatric patients contributes to deleterious outcomes among family members, including relationship problems, psychological distress, and physical morbidity. Furthermore, such associations may be moderated by relationship closeness, pain perception, coping, and communication. In general, the available evidence suggests that greater relationship closeness, increased pain communication, and lower communication efficacy are associated with poorer outcomes among family members, whereas accurate perception of pain is associated with positive outcomes. Future research needs to move beyond observational studies toward the development of interventions aimed at addressing the negative consequences of chronic pain on family members. Future research also needs to include greater examination of the potential modifiable risk factors for family members of patients with chronic pain. Once those risk factors are identified, subsequent efforts should be made to target dyads who are at highest risk for adverse outcomes.

Although significant advances have been made over the past several decades, productive expansion of the field requires a detailed examination of specific subgroups and comparisons by patient age, relationship (spouse vs adult children), and caregiver status. Of utmost importance is examining how chronic pain impacts older patients and their relatives in the face of multimorbidity. Next, we acknowledge the limitations of the current evidence base and highlight opportunities for future investigation.

### Patient Age

One major shortcoming of the existing literature has been the lack of differentiation between middle-aged and older adult samples. As is evident from our review, few studies have explicitly examined the effects of pain experienced by geriatric patients on family members. Instead, the studies reviewed simultaneously include middle-aged and older patients, without further comparison between these subgroups and consequences for their relatives. Importantly, middle-aged and older individuals may differ in their perception of the pain experience,[12] physical disability,[11] and emotion regulation.[63,64] Such differences may have important implications for the interpersonal and emotional effects of pain, including dyadic coping and adjustment. Comparisons by age may therefore expose differences that are relevant for clinical practice and interventions tailored to geriatric patients and their relatives.

### Relationship to the Patient

Research examining the effects of later life pain on family members has predominantly focused on spousal samples. Studies have yet to examine whether and how older parents' pain affects their adult offspring, with only one attempt to include adult children to any extent.[65] This gap warrants attention, given that adult children often have extensive contact with older parents[66] and are the largest group providing informal assistance to individuals ages 65 or older.[67] Although a recent theoretic model has proposed several pathways by which pain in older relatives may affect adult offspring,[68] empirical investigations have yet to surface.

Importantly, the consequences of geriatric patients' pain on adult children may differ from the effects on spouses. Such differences may be examined in light of social structural norms of reciprocity and exchange. According to social exchange theory, adult child caregivers may experience less psychological distress and burden than spouses because providing care to an older parent may be perceived as reciprocation of parents' love and care during childhood.[69] In keeping with this hypothesis, a recent meta-analysis focusing predominantly on caregivers of patients with dementia found that spousal caregivers report more depressive symptoms, greater financial and physical burden, and lower levels of psychological well-being than adult children, but not more emotional burden or social strain.[70] An important contribution to the pain literature would be to make such comparisons among spouses and adult children of geriatric pain sufferers to understand whether and how such differences manifest in this context.

### Caregiver Status

Family caregiving is traditionally defined as providing assistance to a loved one with physical or psychological impairment.[10] Recent reviews of the caregiving literature point to the detrimental impact of care provision on family relationships[71] and caregivers' emotional well-being.[72,73] Compared with noncaregivers, caregivers report greater levels of depression and heightened stress.[74] Both theory and research suggest that increased exposure to the suffering of a loved one may place caregivers at heightened risk of adverse outcomes, above and beyond the physical demands of care provision.[57] Although pain studies have not examined this directly, our review suggests that exposure to frequent pain communication may contribute to poorer marital quality[27] and compromised psychological well-being among relatives.[56] A potential avenue for research would be to examine whether caregivers of geriatric pain patients experience poorer outcomes as compared with noncaregivers, and furthermore, whether these hypothesized differences vary by the quality or frequency of contact between the relative and the pain sufferer.

### Chronic Pain and Multimorbidity

Several studies have identified strong associations between the presence of chronic pain and other chronic illnesses,[13] mental health issues,[75,76] and sleep disorders.[77] Indeed, managing the competing demands of multiple chronic conditions is a significant challenge for many older adults and their family members.[78] However, it remains unclear how older patients and their relatives make treatment choices and manage chronic pain in the face of multiple health conditions. Another important line of research is to investigate whether and how the presence of multimorbidity differentially affects older patients with chronic pain and their caregivers. Moreover, a thorough understanding of this area is essential for developing tailored interventions that address the complex concerns of patients with chronic pain and other chronic conditions and their family members.

## PRACTICE RECOMMENDATIONS

Until clearer evidence becomes available regarding specific approaches to improve outcomes for family members of patients with chronic pain, it is difficult to issue concrete recommendations for practice. Therefore, the recommendations that follow should be viewed within the context of the limited evidence base described previously.

Health care providers should be aware that chronic pain may have an impact on older patients and their family members, and should therefore take a dyadic approach to the assessment of possible adverse outcomes on both individuals. Specifically, health care providers should consider asking older patients with chronic pain and their loved ones about whether and how the patients' pain impacts their interpersonal relationships. For spousal dyads, one approach is to ask patients and their partners about their marital adjustment by using open-ended questions (eg, "In what ways has your pain affected your relationship with your spouse?") or validated instruments, such as the Dyadic Adjustment Scale[79] or Marital Adjustment Test.[80] Whereas open-ended questions may afford an opportunity for patients and their loved ones to discuss a range of issues, standardized tools may help clinicians to quickly identify specific areas of concern.

Providers should also be aware that patients with pain and their family members are susceptible to psychological distress, and should therefore assess for the presence (or absence) of these symptoms in both individuals. Research studies have typically used the Mood and Anxiety Symptom Questionnaire[81] and the Center for Epidemiologic Studies-Depression Scale[82] to assess psychological functioning. These instruments show good discriminant validity and reliability and could be readily applied in clinical practice. The 10-item Perceived Stress Scale has also been used with patients suffering from chronic pain and their relatives.[83] This scale asks respondents to report how uncontrollable, overloaded, and unpredictable their lives have been over the past month. Given that high stress levels are associated with physical morbidities, including elevated blood pressure and susceptibility to infection,[84] this scale may provide additional utility in identifying individuals who may also be at risk of diminished physical health.

Although several family-oriented programs have been developed for patients with chronic pain,[85] interventions that directly address the effects of chronic pain on family members have yet to emerge. It is therefore not possible to recommend specific programs or therapies to address the negative consequences of pain on relatives. To supplement patients' treatment, clinicians may wish to direct family members to the resources and publications available through the National Institute on Aging,[86] American Chronic Pain Association,[87] and National Center on Caregiving.[88] The National Institute on Aging and American Chronic Pain Association Web sites provide links to local support groups for patients and family caregivers and offer educational materials describing the common myths and misunderstandings about pain. The National Center on Caregiving offers a variety of resources, including a state-by-state resource locator to help caregivers connect with others, a research registry for individuals who wish to participate in clinical trials, and a series of instructive webinars designed to help caregivers to manage their stress, communicate more effectively with their loved one and with providers, and learn about new legislation and programs that explicitly address their needs.

## SUMMARY

This review summarizes the existing literature examining the effects of geriatric patients' pain on family members' relationship satisfaction, psychological distress, and physical health. Particular consideration was given to the mechanisms underlying these associations and the theoretic explanations for specific outcomes. Despite growing interest in studying the impact of geriatric pain on family members, understanding of this topic is far from complete. Questions remain about whether the associations between geriatric patients' pain and family members' outcomes differ by patient age, relationship to the patient, and caregiver status. Future research is also needed to determine how families cope with chronic pain within the context of multimorbidity, and to identify the modifiable risk factors for family members. As progress is made on each of these issues, family-based interventions designed for geriatric pain patients and their relatives may play an important role in minimizing relationship discord and improving psychological and physical outcomes.

## REFERENCES

1. Keefe FJ, Somers TJ. Psychological approaches to understanding and treating arthritis pain. Nat Rev Rheumatol 2010;6:210–6.
2. Martire LM, Schulz R, Helgeson VS, et al. Review and meta-analysis of couple-oriented interventions for chronic illness. Ann Behav Med 2010;40(3):325–42.
3. Martire LM. The "relative" efficacy of involving family in psychosocial interventions for chronic illness: are there added benefits to patients and family members? Fam Syst Health 2005;23(3):312–28.
4. Wilson S, Martire LM, Keefe FJ, et al. Daily verbal and nonverbal expression of osteoarthritis pain and spouse responses. Pain 2013;154(10):2045–53.
5. Institute of Medicine. Relieving pain in America: a blueprint for transforming prevention, care, education, and research. Washington, DC: The National Academies Press; 2011.
6. McCarberg BH, Stanos S, Williams DA. Comprehensive chronic pain management: improving physical and psychological function. Am J Med 2012;125(6):S1.
7. Thomas E, Peat G, Harris L, et al. The prevalence of pain and pain interference in a general population of older adults: cross-sectional findings from the North Staffordshire Osteoarthritis Project (NorStOP). Pain 2004;110(1):361–8.
8. Lawrence RC, Felson DT, Helmick CG, et al. Estimates of the prevalence of arthritis and other rheumatic conditions in the United States: Part II. Arthritis Rheumatol 2008;58(1):26–35.
9. Freburger JK, Holmes GM, Agans RP, et al. The rising prevalence of chronic low back pain. Arch Intern Med 2009;169(3):251–8.
10. Talley RC, Crews JE. Framing the public health of caregiving. Am J Public Health 2007;97:224–8.
11. National Institutes of Health. Fact sheet: disability in older adults 2010. NIH RePORT.
12. Gibson SJ, Helme RD. Age-related differences in pain perception and report. Clin Geriatr Med 2001;17(3):433–56.
13. Butchart A, Kerr EA, Heisler M, et al. Experience and management of chronic pain among patients with other complex chronic conditions. Clin J Pain 2009; 25(4):293–8.
14. Kerns RD, Turk DC. Depression and chronic pain: the mediating role of the spouse. J Marriage Fam 1984;46(4):845–52.
15. Leonard MT, Cano A, Johansen AB. Chronic pain in a couples context: a review and integration of theoretical models and empirical evidence. J Pain 2006;7: 377–90.
16. Rosland AM, Heisler M, Piette JD. The impact of family behaviors and communication patterns on chronic illness outcomes: a systematic review. J Behav Med 2010;35(2):221–39.
17. Cano A. Pain catastrophizing and social support in married individuals with chronic pain: the moderating role of pain duration. Pain 2004;110(3):656–64.
18. Romano JM, Turner JA, Jensen MP. The family environment in chronic pain patients: comparison to controls and relationship to patient functioning. J Clin Psychol Med Settings 1997;4:383–95.

19. Romano JM, Turner JA, Clancy SL. Sex differences in the relationship of pain patient dysfunction to spouse adjustment. Pain 1989;39:289–95.

20. Matheson L, Harcourt D, Hewlett S. 'Your whole life, your whole world, it changes': partners' experiences of living with rheumatoid arthritis. Musculoskel Care 2010; 8(1):46–54.

21. Block AR, Kremer E, Gaylor M. Behavioral treatment of chronic pain: the spouse as a discriminative cue for pain behavior. Pain 1980;9:243–52.

22. West C, Usher K, Foster K, et al. Chronic pain and the family: the experience of the partners of people living with chronic pain. J Clin Nurs 2012;21(23–24): 3352–60.

23. Smith AA. Intimacy and family relationships of women with chronic pain. Pain Manag Nurs 2003;4(3):134–42.

24. Flor H, Turk DC, Scholz B. Impact of chronic pain on the spouse: marital, emotional and physical consequences. J Psychosom Res 1987;31:63–71.

25. Schlesinger L. Chronic pain, intimacy, and sexuality: a qualitative study of women who live with pain. J Sex Res 1996;33(3):249–56.

26. Turk DC, Flor H, Rudy TE. Pain and families. I. Etiology, maintenance, and psychosocial impact. Pain 1987;30:3–27.

27. Patterson JM, Garwick AW. The impact of chronic illness on families: a family systems perspective. Ann Behav Med 1994;16:131–42.

28. Cano A, Johansen AB, Leonard MT, et al. What are the marital problems of patients with chronic pain? Curr Pain Headache Rep 2005;9(2):96–100.

29. Smith A, Friedemann ML. Perceived family dynamics of persons with chronic pain. J Adv Nurs 1999;30(3):543–51.

30. Martire LM, Keefe FJ, Schulz R, et al. Older spouses' perceptions of partners' chronic arthritis pain: implications for spousal responses, support provision, and caregiving experiences. Psychol Aging 2006;21:222–30.

31. Riemsma RP, Taal E, Rasker JJ. Perceptions about perceived functional disabilities and pain of people with rheumatoid arthritis: differences between patients and their spouses and correlates with well-being. Arthritis Care Res 2000;13: 255–61.

32. Cano A, Johansen AB, Geisser M. Spousal congruence on disability, pain, and spouse responses to pain. Pain 2004;109(3):258–65.

33. Thompson SC, Pitts JS. In sickness and in health: chronic illness, marriage, and spousal caregiving. In: Spaceman S, Oskamp S, editors. Helping and being helped: naturalistic studies. Newbury Park (CA): Sage Publications; 1992. p. 115–51.

34. Berg CA, Upchurch R. A developmental-contextual model of couples coping with chronic illness across the adult life span. Psychol Bull 2007;133:920–54.

35. Sullivan MJ, Tripp D, Santor D. Gender differences in pain and pain behavior: the role of catastrophizing. Cognit Ther Res 2000;24:121–34.

36. Sullivan MJ. The communal coping model of pain catastrophising: clinical and research implications. Can Psychol 2012;53(1):32–41.

37. Lackner JM, Gurtman MB. Pain catastrophizing and interpersonal problems: a circumplex analysis of the communal coping model. Pain 2004;110(3):597–604.

38. Feinauer L, Steele WR. Caretaker marriages: the impact of chronic pain syndrome on marital adjustment. Am J Fam Ther 1992;20:218–26.

39. Turk DC, Kerns RD. The family in health and illness. In: Turk DC, Kerns RD, editors. Health, illness and families: a life span perspective. New York: Wiley; 1985. p. 1–22.

40. Otis JD, Cardella LA, Kerns RD. The influence of family and culture on pain. Prog Pain Res Manag 2004;27:29–46.

41. Keefe F, Caldwell DS, Baucom D, et al. Spouse-assisted coping skills training in the management of osteoarthritic knee pain. Arthritis Care Res 1996;9(4):279–91.

42. Keefe FJ, Caldwell DS, Baucom D, et al. Spouse-assisted coping skills training in the management of knee pain in osteoarthritis: longterm follow-up results. Arthritis Care Res 1999;12:101–11.

43. Bermas BL, Tucker JS, Winkelman DK, et al. Marital satisfaction in couples with rheumatoid arthritis. Arthritis Care Res 2000;13:149–55.

44. Pennebaker JW, Zech E, Rimé B. Disclosing and sharing emotion: psychological, social, and health consequences. Handbook of bereavement research: consequences, coping, and care. Washington, DC: American Psychological Association; 2001. p. 517–43.

45. Keefe FJ, Smith SJ, Buffington AL, et al. Recent advances and future directions in the biopsychosocial assessment and treatment of arthritis. J Consult Clin Psychol 2002;70(3):640.

46. Fordyce WE. Behavioral methods for chronic pain and illness. St Louis (MO): Mosby; 1976.

47. Craig KD, Versloot J, Goubert L, et al. Perceiving pain in others: automatic and controlled mechanisms. J Pain 2010;11(2):101–8.

48. Cano A, Williams AC. Social interaction in pain: reinforcing pain behaviors or building intimacy? Pain 2010;149(1):9–11.

49. Leonard MT, Cano A. Pain affects spouses too: personal experience with pain and catastrophizing as correlates of spouse distress. Pain 2006;126:139–46.

50. Cunningham MR. Personality and the structure of the nonverbal communication of emotion. J Pers 1977;45:564–83.

51. Hall JA. Gender effects in decoding nonverbal cues. Psychol Bull 1978;85: 845–57.

52. Robinson ME, Wise EA. Gender bias in the observation of experimental pain. Pain 2003;104(1):259–64.

53. Newton-John TR, Williams AC. Chronic pain couples: perceived marital interactions and pain behaviours. Pain 2006;123(1):53–63.

54. Schwartz L, Slater MA, Birchler GR, et al. Depression in spouses of chronic pain patients: the role of patient pain and anger, and marital satisfaction. Pain 1991; 44(1):61–7.

55. Stephens MAP, Martire LM, Cremeans-Smith JK, et al. Older women with osteoarthritis and their caregiving husbands: effects of pain and pain expression on husbands' well-being and support. Rehabil Psychol 2006;51(1):3–12.

56. Druley JA, Stephens MAP, Martire LM, et al. Emotional congruence in older couples coping with wives' osteoarthritis: exacerbating effects of pain behavior. Psychol Aging 2003;18(3):406–14.

57. Monin JK, Schulz R. Interpersonal effects of suffering in older adult caregiving relationships. Psychol Aging 2009;24(3):681–95.

58. Polenick CA, Martire LM, Hemphill RC, et al. Effects of change in arthritis severity on spouse well-being: the moderating role of relationship closeness. J Fam Psychol 2015;29(3):331.

59. Porter LS, Keefe FJ, Wellington C, et al. Pain communication in the context of osteoarthritis: patient and partner self-efficacy for pain communication and holding back from discussion of pain and arthritis-related concerns. Clin J Pain 2008; 24(8):662–8.

60. Rowat K, Knafl KA. Living with chronic pain: the spouse's perspective. Pain 1985; 23(3):259–71.

61. Bigatti S, Cronan T. An examination of the physical health, health care use, and psychological well-being of spouses of people with fibromyalgia syndrome. Health Psychol 2002;21:157–66.

62. Martire LM, Keefe FJ, Schulz R, et al. The impact of daily arthritis pain on spouse sleep. Pain 2013;154(9):1725–31.

63. Charles ST. Strength and vulnerability integration: a model of emotional well-being across adulthood. Psychol Bull 2010;136:1068–91.

64. Urry HL, Gross JJ. Emotion regulation in older age. Curr Dir Psychol Sci 2010;19: 352–7.

65. Hsu KY, Tsai YF, Lin P, et al. Primary family caregivers' observations and perceptions of their older relatives' knee osteoarthritis pain and pain management: a qualitative study. J Adv Nurs 2015;71(9):2119–28.

66. Fingerman KL, Pillemer KA, Silverstein M, et al. The Baby Boomers' intergenerational relationships. Gerontologist 2011;52:199–209.

67. Center on Aging Society. Informal Caregiver Supplement (ICS) to the 1999 National Longterm Care Survey (NLTCS). Washington, DC: Urban Institute; 1999.

68. Riffin C, Suitor JJ, Reid MC, et al. Chronic pain and parent–child relations in later life: an important, but understudied issue. Fam Sci 2012;3(2):75–85.

69. Wright DL, Aquilino WS. Influence of emotional support exchange in marriage on caregiving wives' burden and marital satisfaction. Fam Relat 1998;47:195–204.

70. Pinquart M, Sörensen S. Spouses, adult children, and children-in-law as caregivers of older adults: a meta-analytic comparison. Psychol Aging 2011;26(1):1.

71. Quinn C, Clare L, Woods B. The impact of the quality of relationship on the experiences and wellbeing of caregivers of people with dementia: a systematic review. Aging Ment Health 2009;13(2):143–54.

72. Cuijpers P. Depressive disorders in caregivers of dementia patients: a systematic review. Aging Ment Health 2005;9(4):325–30.

73. Williams AL, McCorkle R. Cancer family caregivers during the palliative, hospice, and bereavement phases: a review of the descriptive psychosocial literature. Palliat Support Care 2011;9(3):315–25.

74. Gallagher-Thompson D, Dal Canto PG, Jacob T, et al. A comparison of marital interaction patterns between couples in which the husband does or does not have Alzheimer's disease. J Gerontol B Psychol Sci Soc Sci 2001;56(3):S140–50.

75. Bair MJ, Robinson RL, Katon W, et al. Depression and pain comorbidity: a literature review. Arch Intern Med 2003;163(20):2433–45.

76. Sareen J, Cox BJ, Clara I, et al. The relationship between anxiety disorders and physical disorders in the US National Comorbidity Survey. Depress Anxiety 2005; 21(4):193–202.

77. Ohayon MM. Relationship between chronic painful physical condition and insomnia. J Psychiatr Res 2005;39(2):151–9.

78. Wolff JL, Starfield B, Anderson G. Prevalence, expenditures, and complications of multiple chronic conditions in the elderly. Arch Intern Med 2002;162(20): 2269–76.

79. Gottman JM, Krakoff LJ. Marital interaction and satisfaction: a longitudinal view. J Consult Clin Psychol 1989;57:47–52.

80. Locke H, Wallace K. Short marital-adjustment and prediction tests: their reliability and validity. Marriage Fam Living 1959;21:251–5.

81. Watson D, Weber K, Assenheimer JS, et al. Testing a tripartite model: I. Evaluating the convergent and discriminant validity of anxiety and depression symptoms scales. J Abnorm Psychol 1995;104:3–14.

82. Radloff LS. The CES–D Scale: a self-report depression scale for research in the general population. Appl Psychol Meas 1977;1:385–401.

83. Cohen S, Karamark T, Mermelstien R. A global measure of perceived stress. J Health Soc Behav 1983;24:385–96.

84. Cohen S, Frank E, Doyle WJ, et al. Types of stressors that increase susceptibility to the common cold in healthy adults. Health Psychol 1998;17:214–23.

85. Riffin C, Pillemer K, Reid MC. Caring for individuals suffering from chronic pain. In: Burgio LD, Gangler JE, Algare DI, editors. The Oxford University Edited Volume: the spectrum of family caregiving for adults and elders with chronic conditions. New York: Oxford University Press; 2015.

86. AgePage. Pain: You can get help. National Institute on Aging. National Institutes of Health. 2015. p. 1–14. Available at: https://www.nia.nih.gov/health/publication/pain. Accessed January 5, 2016.

87. Pain Management Tools. American Chronic Pain Association. 2015. Available at: theapca.org. Accessed January 5, 2016.

88. Taking Care of YOU: Self-Care for Family Caregivers. Family Caregiver Alliance (National Center on Caregiving). 2015. Available at: https://www.caregiver.org/taking-care-you-self-care-family-caregivers. Accessed January 5, 2016.

# Assessment and Measurement of Pain in Adults in Later Life

Staja Q. Booker, MS, RN[1], Keela A. Herr, PhD, RN*

## KEYWORDS

- Aging • Assessment • Later life • Measurement • Older adult • Pain • Self-report

## KEY POINTS

- Pain is a common health issue experienced by adults in their later years.
- Assessment, reassessment, and measurement of pain requires a consistent approach, and is critical to the pain management plan.
- Self-report is the key component and practice standard for assessment of pain presence, intensity, and interference and should be obtained from all older adults when possible.
- Sensory, motor, and cognitive impairments along with language issues can affect an older adults' ability and reliability to provide a timely and accurate self-report of pain.
- Assessment of pain should include developing goals for comfort, function, and mood.

## INTRODUCTION

Pain is a complex, multifaceted problem for aging adults who make up a moderate proportion of persistent pain sufferers. Knowing that many older adults experience pain warrants pain vigilance by providers who are expected to regularly assess pain and provide timely interventions when needed. However, older adults are significantly less likely to have any pain assessment or reassessment documented,[1,2] which contributes to undertreatment. A systematic or step-by-step approach is recommended.[3,4] This article describes a focused pain assessment for the older adult able to provide a reliable report of pain (**Table 1** ).[5] Readers interested in learning more about the components of a comprehensive pain assessment should read Malec and Shega's[6] recent review on this topic.

Disclosure Statement: The authors have nothing to disclose.

The University of Iowa, College of Nursing, 50 Newton Road, Iowa City, IA 52242, USA

[1] 415 Northeast Street, Jonesboro, LA 71251.

* Corresponding author. The University of Iowa, College of Nursing, 50 Newton Road, 306 CNB, Iowa City, IA 52242.

E-mail address: keela-herr@uiowa.edu

| Table 1 | | |
| --- | --- | --- |
| Steps for a focused pain assessment in older adults | | |
| Step | Cognitively Intact and/or Able to Self-Report | Cognitively Impaired and/or Unable to Self-Report |
| 1 | Determine ability to reliably self-report pain and attempt to obtain self-report. | Same as for those able to self-report. Also note if there is a diagnosis of cognitive impairment or dementia. If able to self-report, continue with steps 2–6 in the left column. If unable to self-report, continue with steps 2–6 below. |
| 2 | Determine presence or absence of pain by asking older adult if she or he is experiencing pain, hurt, aches, or discomfort "right now" or "at this moment." | Search for possible causes/sources of pain. |
| 3 | Measure self-reported pain intensity using a valid, reliable, and preferred pain scale, such as the Faces Pain Rating Scale–revised, Iowa Pain Thermometer, and Verbal Descriptor Scale. | Observe for potential pain behaviors using reliable and valid pain–behavior observation tool. |
| 4 | Assess impact of pain on function to determine pain tolerability. | Incorporate proxy reporting. |
| 5 | Assess interference of pain on sleep and emotional stability. | Initiate analgesic trial to evaluate if pain is the cause of behaviors. |
| 6 | Develop a multimodal plan of pain care with realistic goals for comfort, function, and mood. | If the analgesic trial confirms pain, develop a multimodal plan of pain care evaluating treatment options' risks/benefits. |

Courtesy of S. Booker, MS, RN, PhD(c) and K.A. Herr, PhD, RN, FAAN, University of Iowa, College of Nursing, 2015.

## PAIN ASSESSMENT
### Importance of Assessment

A considerable number of community-dwelling and facility-dwelling (ie, nursing homes) older adults experience persistent pain. Approximately 65% of cognitively intact community-dwelling older adults report pain in the last 3 months,[7] and similarly, 63.5% of adults with cognitive impairment report bothersome pain.[8] Pimentel and colleagues[9] found that 65% of nursing homes residents with cancer had pain, with slightly more than 60% having moderate pain and 13.5% severe pain. More concerning, however, is that an unacceptable number of older adults are not prescribed nondrug interventions[10] nor are taking analgesic medications.[8,9] With such a large number of older adults in pain and undertreated, it is imperative that pain is assessed regularly, based on the type of pain, severity and impact of pain and setting of care, and appropriate treatment provided. Although numerous barriers are cited for under-assessment and decreased self-report,[11] it is unacceptable that pain assessment remains incomplete, undocumented, and non–evidence-based across health care settings despite its designation as the fifth vital sign. The intent of the "fifth vital sign" was to encourage providers and nurses to assess pain more frequently and comprehensively. Since this designation, some studies show modest improvement in assessment,[12] whereas others show that pain assessment in older adults remains low and inconsistently documented in patient medical records in acute care.[2] This is likely owing to a continued need for more provider education on the meaning and effective implementation of pain as the fifth vital sign.

Some providers may believe that, because an older adult is known to have persistent pain, there is no need to assess pain but to simply provide treatments. This is haphazard and potentially harmful because an older adult may experience an acute episode of pain in addition to persistent pain (also known as acute-on-chronic pain or acute pain superimposed on chronic pain), and timely assessment could identify any urgent pain problems, as well as be used to tailor the treatment plan. However, recent research shows that treatment of pain in older adults is associated with pain type; for example, abdominal pain is treated with less analgesics as compared with pain owing to fractures.[13] Continued efforts are needed to ensure not only regular and appropriate assessment of pain in older adults, but the essential follow-up in developing and implementing an effective treatment plan.

### Types and causes of pain

The prevalence of persistent pain increases in later life owing to chronic diseases, acute injuries, and cancer. Abdominal pain and fractures are the 2 most common reasons for older adults presenting to the emergency department.[13] Often older adults have complex chronic health conditions that result in multiple etiologies of acute and persistent pain. Persistent pain may be a chronic disease unto itself or a symptom of a chronic disease or acute illness. Common pain types and conditions in older adults are provided below:

- Nociceptive – *somatic*: arthritis, gout, chronic low back pain, thermal (cold or heat) burns, pressure ulcers and wounds, skin rashes, fractures
- Nociceptive – *visceral*: pleurisy, diverticulitis, constipation, gastrointestinal ulcers
- Neuropathic – *central*: phantom limb pain, poststroke pain syndrome
- Neuropathic – *peripheral*: diabetic neuropathy, shingles, postherpetic neuralgia
- Mixed and undetermined: cancer, fibromyalgia, polymyalgia, rheumatic, headaches, mental health disorders (eg, depression, posttraumatic stress disorder)

Pain that goes untreated or undertreated has a high likelihood of causing detrimental consequences, such as pain homeostenosis,[14] functional decline, incapacitation, and frailty.[6,15] Pain assessment from a prevention perspective should be given as much attention as other primary preventive actions, such as vaccinations, in older adults.

### Initiation of Pain Assessment

When and who should assess pain are often asked questions by providers. Determining the interval at which pain is assessed should occur preferably during the first interaction with the patient, but will vary depending on severity of pain, the type of institution, and needs of the patient. For example, it is crucial that older adults are screened for pain before a procedure to establish a baseline, identify those at high risk for developing persistent postsurgical pain, and determine if perioperative accommodations such as positioning or use of intraoperative analgesics are needed. After the procedure, pain should be reassessed promptly, keeping in mind that the older adult postsedation may have difficulty understanding pain questioning and articulating a reliable answer. In long-term care, pain assessment may be conducted daily, weekly, or quarterly to identify new pain problems and monitor persistent pain problems.

All health care providers play key roles in assessment of pain: the primary care provider/hospitalist, nurse, nursing assistant, rehabilitative and respiratory therapists, and social workers. The main points to consider with interdisciplinary pain assessment is that everyone uses a consistent approach and same pain scale, documents the assessment in an accessible location, and communicates their findings to other team members.

### Intent of Assessment

Self-report is the single most reliable method to determine experience of pain; other methods, such as nurse report or proxy report, are fraught with limitations usually resulting in underestimation or overestimation of pain or little agreement with patient self-report.[16–18] Self-report is recognized as the gold standard for measuring pain in clinical practice and research.[18] Patient reports are the primary source of information on pain presence, intensity, and impact/interference on daily life. The pain assessment process should always begin with an attempt to obtain a verbal (or nonverbal, namely, deliberate hand gestures, head nods, hand shake) self-report of pain from all older adults, even those with cognitive impairment.[18] Although seemingly a simple task, providers frequently neglect to ask older adults about pain despite agreement that consistent assessment is an essential component for good pain management. Cognitive, sensory, and communication impairments present challenges to assessment of pain in older adults. These impairments may necessitate proxy report from family or caregivers to help gather self-report or to confirm pain.

#### Challenges in obtaining self-report

Cognitive impairment is single-handedly one of the most prevalent barriers noted by providers, and many assume that those with cognitive impairment are unable to respond to pain questions and provide self-report. Older adults with cognitive impairments may have difficulty verbally describing their pain experiences, but research clearly shows that cognitive impairment and dementia do not always limit self-report.[18–20] In assessing the presence of pain, there was moderate agreement between self-report of pain and use of a nonverbal observational pain scale in older adults with cognitive impairment.[17] Therefore, it is important to determine the older adult's ability and reliability to provide an accurate report of pain by using one of the techniques in **Table 2** (column 1).[22–25] When cognition or memory is affected, family or caregivers can provide information on pain. Although cognition itself cannot be acutely improved, the methods used to assess pain can be simplified to enhance patient understanding and obtain patient self-report. When reliability of self-report is suspect, if available, proxy reporters (eg, family, certified nursing assistants) should be used to identify the presence or absence of pain. Studies support accurate recognition of pain presence, but proxy reporters are not reliable estimators of pain severity.[26]

Providers should assess for and address any sensory and language barriers. Sensory impairments in hearing, vision, and speech can impede pain assessment. Older adults with hearing impairments may not hear the question being asked or may not hear the question accurately, thus providing an answer that is not reliable. Hearing aids or amplifiers should be in place before pain conversation with the older adult. When vision is impaired, the older adult may be unable to see a pain scale on paper or mobile device. Communicating with deaf older adults is another issue that has not been adequately addressed. In these cases, a sign language interpreter or communication tool should be used. Explaining the appearance of the scale can help older adults to visualize the scale and choose an appropriate rating. Motor impairments may limit an older adult's ability to use purposeful nonverbal methods of communication (eg, pointing finger to a number or face on a pain scale or hand squeezes to reply yes/no to pain question). Booker and Haedtke[4] provide a table on how to address sensory impairments in older adults when conducting a pain assessment.

Tools translated and validated for culturally diverse patients and a translator or communication tool should be available when assessing pain in any adult.[18] The Faces Pain Scale-revised (described elsewhere in this paper) does not require reading or writing ability; thus, the tool may be useful for non–English-speaking older adults.[18] Once cognitive, sensory, and communication barriers are addressed, providers should use a self-report approach to assess pain. Self-report approaches can be general or condition specific and will depend on the willingness of the older adult to openly discuss pain.

### General self-report approach: pain presence

The most common and general approach to identifying pain is to simply ask older adults by obtaining self-report. Acute pain may prompt self-report more readily than pain that is constant or persistent. When gathering self-report from older adults, providers should prompt simple and concrete questions (eg, "Does this hurt?").[27] A common mistake made by providers when obtaining self-report is to ask "How are you doing?" or "Are you comfortable?" to solicit a response about pain. Questions about general well-being should not be substituted for pain assessment because these may elicit socially desirable answers and may not elicit any information about pain.[4,18] Instead questions should explicitly ask about pain or hurt. Although a question such as "How are you feeling?" or "How did you sleep last night?" can elicit information on pain and pain interference from some older adults, for others, this question could represent their affect or mood as opposed to pain. When an older adult uses these questions as an opportunity to report pain, providers should then explore in more detail the characteristics of pain (ie, intensity, location, duration).

Pain assessment is an interactive and collaborative process[28] and frequently requires creative adaptation to obtain patient self-report. Ensuring privacy can help to elicit an open and honest self-report. Older adults may need repeated explanations about the pain assessment tool and a longer time to respond. Denial or minimization of pain is common among older adults, and they may fear the consequences of acknowledging pain (eg, extensive tests/procedures, retaliation from providers). When denial or minimization of pain occurs, it is recommended that the pain question be rephrased using pain synonyms or use an open-ended question. Open-ended questions or statements generally provide a better response, and opens the conversation to allow the older adult to explain the pain in their words.[29] Examples of open-ended questions are, "Please, tell me about your pain (aches or soreness)." Close-ended or biased questions, such as "You aren't in any pain, are you?" will likely not elicit true responses from older adults. Another technique that may prove effective in garnering self-report is to assess pain at specific times of the day. For example, a provider might assess pain in an older adult with osteoarthritis early in the morning or shortly after awakening.

### Condition-specific self-report approach: pain presence

When older adults do not self-report pain during general questioning, but pain is highly suspected, a more focused approach can be helpful. A "where does it hurt" approach asks specifically about body locations (ie, pain extensity), possible conditions, or medical procedures that could cause pain. This is a helpful technique for acute care when pain may be more localized owing to injury or procedures. For example, if the medical history notes a diagnosis of osteoarthritis of the knees, then providers should ask older adults specifically about any current pain in their knees. Knowing medical diagnoses,

**Table 2**
Pain self-report determination and tool selection process

| Reliability and Ability to Self-Report Determination Process[4] | Pain Tool Selection Process[24] | | Additional Considerations for Pain Tool Selection[4] |
|---|---|---|---|
| Triggers to establish self-report ability: Note a diagnosis of cognitive impairment, dementia, or mental health condition, Note a condition that may interfere with verbal report (eg, aphasia), Administer a quick, reliable mental status examination, and/or Observe coherence of thoughts and verbal communication (and/or ability to explain what pain is to them). Techniques to establish reliability to self-report using pain tools: Ask older adult to pick 2 words that similarly describe pain from a list mixed with pain and nonpain descriptors and observe for conceptual understanding. | If older adult: Can communicate verbally or nonverbally purposefully (eg, pointing, head nods, etc.), can self-report reliably, and is cognitively intact. | ⬆ Use a valid, reliable, and patient-preferred self-report pain scale such as: • FPS-r • VDS • IPT-r • NRS | Congruent with patient's culture of pain expression, accurate language, and available in different languages (or can be easily translated). Accommodates patient's sensory impairments. Accommodates patient's developmental, intellectual, and cognitive level; easily understood. Easily and quickly explained to patient or observer. Easily used, scored, and recorded consistently. Can be used by interdisciplinary personnel. Easily linked to patient's comfort–function–mood goals. Meets organizational and regulatory standards. Fits with quality indicators and institutional documentation system. |
| | Cannot consistently communicate verbally or nonverbally purposefully, cannot self-report consistently, and has fluctuating cognitive status (eg, dementia, delirium). | ⬆ Attempt self-report first by using a valid, reliable, and preferred self-report pain scale (see previous) and observational pain–behavior tool such as: • PAINAD • PACSLAC-II • Abbey Pain Scale • DOLOPLUS-2 | |
| | Cannot communicate verbally, cannot self-report, and is not cognitively intact. | ⬆ Use an assessment protocol such as the: • Hierarchy of Pain Assessment[25] • ADD[26] • MOBID-2 and a valid, reliable observational pain–behavior tool (see previous). | |

Assess conceptual understanding on the use of a self-report pain scale by asking the person where mild and severe pain are represented on a 0–10 pain scale, then repeat this task several minutes later (should have the same or similar scores if reliably reporting pain)[18]. this can also be done by asking if 7 is more intense pain than 9 on the NRS.

Use a pain screener test.[21]

Can be used as data for quality improvement and evidence-based practice projects.

*Abbreviations:* ADD, Assessment of Discomfort in Dementia Protocol; FPS-r, Faces Pain Scale-revised; IPT-r, Iowa Pain Thermometer-revised; MOBID-2, Mobilization-Observation-Behavior-Intensity-Dementia-2 pain scale; NRS, Numeric Rating Scale; PACSLAC-II, Pain Assessment Checklist for Seniors with Limited Ability to Communicate; PAINAD, Pain Assessment in Advanced Dementia; VDS, Verbal Descriptor Scale.

*Courtesy of* S. Booker, MS, RN, PhD(c) and K.A. Herr, PhD, RN, FAAN, University of Iowa, College of Nursing. 2015; and *Data from* Refs.[22–25]

the admitting issues, or recent trauma can influence the specificity of pain questions. If the older adult has had recent trauma, it is good to frame pain screening questions based on this history. For example, "You had a hard fall today; do you hurt or have any soreness anywhere (or *a specific location*)?" This condition-specific approach acknowledges the potential pain-causing condition and reinforces the notion that older adults' pain is important to know about and control.

The condition-specific approach is not without limitations. The pain communication of an older adult is influenced by their cultural and generational language. For example, a provider may ask "Do you have a headache?", but an older adult may respond differently to "Does your head ache?" Herr[18] recommends documenting the language or descriptors that older adults use to describe pain, and then providers using the patient's same language in subsequent assessments.

A different approach is to provide a body map to the older adult and ask him or her to point or mark the area where they are hurting or having pain. A picture communication pain tool originally developed for children, the Mesko-Eliades Pain Area Locator Tool,[30] may have promise for use in older adults. Other simple body maps can also work, for example, the Brief Pain Inventory–Short Form (BPI-SF) includes a body map.[31] Not only do older adults provide key information about the location of pain using this approach but also the presence of pain.

### Proxy report to support self-report

Although older adults with cognitive, intellectual, and communication impairments may be able to report pain, proxy informants like family and caregivers can provide additional information about whether a patient does or does not have pain. Proxies (or surrogates) can discuss with providers more details about pain that the older adult is unable to articulate clearly, these being, location and duration of pain, effectiveness of pain treatment, and relevant medical history. Proxies should, however, be someone who has intimate knowledge of the patient's pain history and is trustworthy in helping the older patient manage pain treatment plans, especially when opioids are used. As noted, seeking information about pain from spouses, adult children, or paid caregivers may be helpful to support pain assessment and treatment decisions, but should not supplant self-report that is judged reliable.

In recent years, there has been an explosion of mobile applications that allow patients to record pain ratings and send real-time pain assessments to providers.[32,33] Specifically, there are many applications for arthritis, chronic low back pain, and fibromyalgia where patients can monitor and manage their daily pain. These momentary recordings can be sent to providers in real time or shared with providers at inpatient clinic visits or via telehealth visits. Caregivers can use mobile applications and digital technologies to send proxy report of pain or patients' self-report of pain to the provider to facilitate real-time treatment. Although little evidence is available regarding older adults' use of mobile applications for pain assessment and monitoring, the growing resources and tools are likely to be appropriate for use with those who are technologically savvy and willing to use innovative approaches to communicate with their providers.

### Unidimensional self-report tools: pain intensity and impact

Most unidimensional tools used for focused assessments ask about the severity or intensity of pain and impact of pain on function (**Table 3**).

**Intensity** Professional organizations and geriatric pain experts recommend a quantitative assessment using standardized, reliable pain intensity tools for older adults.[3,18]

**Table 3**
Synthesis of evidence on unidimensional pain intensity self-report scales in older adults

| Scale | Other Names | Scale Orientation | Scale Metrics | Level of Conceptual Understanding Needed | Recommendations |
|---|---|---|---|---|---|
| Colored Analog Scale (CAS) | None | Horizontal or vertical | Uses colors to represent increasing pain; begins with white (no pain) and increases to red (extreme pain). | Minimal-moderate | Can be used in older adults with and without cognitive impairment. Ensure older adult understands what the colors represent. May not be appropriate for all cultures. Visual acuity must be intact. |
| Faces Pain Scale-revised (FPS-R) | None; different from the Wong-Baker FACES scale | Horizontal | 0–10 (Face 1 = 0, Face 2 = 2, Face 3 = 4, Face 4 = 6, Face 5 = 8, Face 6 = 10) | Moderate-significant | Recommended in older adults including ethnic minorities. Clearly explain that faces represent pain and not mood/emotional state. Visual acuity must be intact. |
| Iowa Pain Thermometers (IPT) | Pain thermometers, Iowa Pain Thermometer-revised (IPT-r) | Vertical | Uses a picture of a thermometer with colors similar to CAS, verbal descriptors, and numbers to show increasing pain. IPT: No pain to the most intense pain imaginable. IPT-r: 0–10 and no pain to The most intense pain imaginable. | Minimal | Recommended in older adults including those with cognitive impairment and ethnic minorities. Can gather a numeric and descriptive rating using this scale. Visual acuity must be intact. |

(continued on next page)

| Scale | Other Names | Scale Orientation | Scale Metrics | Level of Conceptual Understanding Needed | Recommendations |
|---|---|---|---|---|---|
| **Table 3** *(continued)* | | | | | |
| Numeric Rating Scale (NRS) | Verbal Numeric Rating Scale (VNRS) | Horizontal or vertical. Can be administered verbally or written. | 0–5, 0–10, 0–20, or 0–100 (0 = No pain and 5, 10, 20, 100 = extreme pain) | Moderate-significant | Use a vertical NRS. Often used in most settings, but may be difficult for older adults with cognitive impairment. |
| Verbal Descriptor Scale (VDS) | Simple Descriptive Scale, Verbal Rating Scale (VRS) | Horizontal or vertical | A combination of any of the following descriptors: no pain, slight pain, minor pain, mild pain, moderate pain, severe pain, very severe pain, extreme pain, pain as bad as it could be, worst imaginable pain, worst possible pain. Usually have 4–6 descriptor anchors. Pain thermometers are an example of a VDS. | Minimal-moderate | Older adults with and without cognitive impairments can use this scale. Ensure verbal descriptors are simple and match patient's cultural language. |
| Visual analog scale | None | Horizontal or vertical | Anchored with no pain and pain as bad as it could be or 0 and 10. | Moderate-significant | Difficult to conceptually understand leading to higher failure rates and low reliability. Avoid in older adults. |

Notes: These scales can be used across setting types, ethnic cultures, and cognitive status.
*Data from* Hadjistavropoulos T, Herr K, Turk DC, et al. An interdisciplinary expert consensus statement on assessment of pain in older persons. Clin J Pain 2007;23(suppl 1):S1–43.

Providers often note the difficulty in selecting an appropriate pain tool for pain intensity, but **Table 2** can assist in tool selection.

The intensity of pain can be described numerically (quantification), descriptively (qualification), or both. Tools using numeric ratings include the Numeric Rating Scale (NRS; 0–10). The simple Verbal Descriptor Scale (VDS) and original Iowa Pain Thermometer (IPT)[34] use words to describe pain severity, whereas the Faces Pain Scale-revised uses facial expressions to simulate increasing pain severity ratings.[35] The IPT-revised (IPT-r) uses both numbers (ie, 0–10) and pain descriptor words, aligned with a thermometer, to help older adults more accurately self-report pain intensity.[36] These measures have been tested in diverse older adult populations, and the Faces Pain Scale-revised, VDS, and IPT-r are the most preferred tools.[36] For older adults with hearing impairments, a visual pain scale, such as the FPS-r, with written instructions may be appropriate; a verbal scale (eg, verbal NRS or VDS) can be used with patients with vision deficits.

Some studies have examined the correlation between numeric pain ratings and verbal descriptors to determine the most effective and patient-preferred method to assess pain intensity. Because pain treatment decisions are often based on determination of mild, moderate or severe pain status, the concordance of tools with varying approaches to assessment with the NRS is useful. According to Edelen and Saliba[37] and Jones and colleagues,[38] item response theory between the VDS and NRS found that older adults with varying cognitive status rated pain as follows:

- No pain = 0 (NRS)
- Mild pain (VDS) = 1 to 4 (NRS)
- Moderate pain (VDS) = 5 to 7 (NRS)
- Severe pain (VDS) = 7 to 10 (NRS)
- Very severe (VDS) = 10 (NRS).

Other studies have also used similar methods to determine cut-offs for mild, moderate, and severe pain. Jones and colleagues[38] compared the VDS with the original Faces Pain Scale and found the following correlations:

- No pain = face 1
- Mild pain (VDS) = faces 2 and 3
- Moderate pain (VDS) = face 4
- Severe pain (VDS) = faces 5, 6, and 7.

**Impact/interference** Pain intensity alone does not provide an adequate picture of pain or its tolerability. Some older adults are, and providers should be, more concerned about how pain impacts their physical and mental function—mobility, mood, fatigue—rather than pain intensity itself.[28] This involves assessing the extent to which pain interferes with daily activities and how tolerable pain is to engage in daily activities. The Functional Pain Scale is a short, self-report tool to gauge how pain interferes with functional ability.[39,40] Another simple strategy includes asking older patients directly in a pain interview about what they cannot do because of pain but want to do.

*Multidimensional self-report tools: Pain intensity and impact*
Several tools used for more comprehensive assessments of pain intensity and impact on and interference with daily function that have been validated for use with older adults include the BPI-SF,[31,41] Geriatric Pain Measure-Short Form,[42] and Pain Intensity, Enjoyment in Life, and General Activity questionnaire.[43] The BPI is one of the most recommended tools, and is useful in identifying older adults at risk for falls due to pain.[44] Undertreated and overtreated pain can impair physical function and mobility

and cause fatigue, all 3 of which significantly increase the risk for falls in aging adults. Assessment should also verify the presence (or absence of) of delirium, sedation, imbalance, or other factors that can inform judgment about pain and potential risk of falls.

Multidimensional tools are particularly useful when conducting comprehensive pain assessments during the first primary care visit, upon admission to a new care setting, and at select intervals in long-term care settings. However, comprehensive tools require a higher level of conceptual understanding than single-item pain tools. Specifically each tool assesses:

- BPI-SF: 15 questions evaluate pain intensity (0–100), interference, and location; pain treatments and relief.
- Geriatric Pain Measure-Short Form: 12 questions ask about pain intensity (mild pain: <30, moderate pain: 30–69, severe pain: ≥70) and interference.
- Pain Intensity, Enjoyment in Life, and General Activity: 3 questions assess pain intensity and interference on enjoyment in life and general activity.

There is a high rate of new or existing moderate to severe pain during care transitions (eg, acute to long-term care setting) in older adults.[45] A modified comprehensive assessment using any of these tools to identify causes, qualities, and severity of pain may be needed at discharge, and this information should be clearly documented and communicated during transitions of care. The presence of pain is demonstrated in cross-setting data from Simmons and colleagues[45] in which 51% of older adults had moderate-to-severe pain before hospitalization, upon hospital discharge (38%), and after admission to a skilled nursing facility (53%).

### Goals for comfort–function–mood

When pain is reported, the assessment process is incomplete if a comfort–function–mood goal is not developed collaboratively between older patient and provider. This biopsychosocial goal guides treatment intervention and reassessment parameters. In terms of comfort, this relates to reducing pain intensity or number of breakthrough pain episodes, achieving a tolerable level of pain, and satisfaction with pain management.[46] Families of older adults reported greater satisfaction with end-of-life comfort care when a comfort goal was developed on admission to the nursing home.[47]

As the evidence base grows, the goals of pain management for older patients are shifting from a focus on decreasing pain intensity to a certain pain level to positively affecting function, whether this is to maintain function or improve pain-related disability. Many older adults simply want pain to be tolerable to remain independent and physically and socially functional. Improving mood and satisfaction with life with persistent pain may also be important goals.

### PAIN REASSESSMENT

Assessment of pain is an iterative and collaborative process, but reassessment of pain is commonly neglected breaching the continuity of pain control.[1] Having a routine order for pain medication should not replace regularly scheduled assessments of pain. In fact, baseline assessment of pain provides a reference point for follow-up assessments when evaluating the effectiveness of the routine treatment or assessing for adverse effects of pharmacologic treatments. Assessment completed over time should use the same pain self-report tool and assessor when possible, and conduct

**Box 1**
**Geriatric pain resources**

- Geriatric pain http://www.geriatricpain.org/Pages/home.aspx
- Hartford Institute for Geriatric Nursing https://consultgeri.org/try-this/general-assessment
  - Modules: Assessing Pain in Older Adults, Assessment of Nociceptive versus Neuropathic Pain in Older Adults, and Assessing Pain in Persons with Dementia
- Collaboration for Home Care Advances in Management and Practice (CHAMP) geriatric pain management course http://www.champ-program.org/page/66/geriatric-pain-management-course
- Health in Aging: "Pain Management" http://www.healthinaging.org/aging-and-health-a-to-z/topic:pain-management/
- City of Hope Pain Resource Center http://prc.coh.org/pain_assessment.asp

pain assessment under similar situations (eg, during movement).[27] Reassessment should always occur:

- Upon transitions of care/settings—discharge and admission
- After initial report of pain, regardless of intervention administration
- At each new report of pain (eg, breakthrough pain)
- After any intervention (pharmacologic, including analgesic trials in nonverbal older adults, and nondrug) has been provided to determine efficacy in reducing pain intensity and/or improving pain-related disability. If a medication is given, reassess at predetermined intervals: (1) at the onset of action of analgesic effect, (2) during the peak analgesic effect, and (3) at the time when medication levels are lowest (ie, generally 4–6 hours after administration).
- Within 6 hours after first acute pain assessment in the emergency department.[48]
- To determine if there is a need to modify comfort–function–mood goals.[46]

## SUMMARY

Advancing age and multiple comorbidities heighten the risk of persistent pain in older adults. Therefore, assessment of persistent and acute pain is an important part of preventative and palliative health care in older adults. Using the techniques discussed in this article can assist providers in assessing pain and obtaining self-report from older adults. **Box 1** provides a list of geriatric pain resources for readers interested in learning more about this topic.

## REFERENCES

1. Herr K, Titler M. Acute pain assessment and pharmacological management practices for the older adult with a hip fracture: a review of ED trends. J Emerg Nurs 2009;35(4):312–20.
2. Spillman SK, Baumhover LA, Lillegraven CL, et al. Infrequent assessment of pain in elderly trauma patients. J Trauma Nurs 2014;21(5):229–35.
3. Hadjistavropoulos T, Herr K, Turk DC, et al. An interdisciplinary expert consensus statement on assessment of pain in older persons. Clin J Pain 2007;23(Suppl 1): S1–43.
4. Booker SQ, Haedtke C. Assessing pain in verbal older adults. Nursing 2016; 46(2):65–8.

5. Booker S, Herr K. Pain in older patients. In: Murinson BB, Barreveld A, editors. Fundamentals of pain care. London: Oxford University Press, in press.

6. Malec M, Shega JW. Pain management in the elderly. Med Clin North Am 2015; 99(2):337–50.

7. Nahin RL. Estimates of pain prevalence and severity in adults: United States, 2012. J Pain 2015;16(8):769–80.

8. Hunt LJ, Covinsky KE, Yaffe K, et al. Pain in community-dwelling older adults with dementia: results from the National Health and Aging Trends study. J Am Geriatr Soc 2015;63(8):1503–11.

9. Pimentel CB, Briesacher BA, Gurwitz JH, et al. Pain management in nursing home residents with cancer. J Am Geriatr Soc 2015;63(4):633–41.

10. Rasu RS, Sohraby R, Cunningham L, et al. Assessing chronic pain treatment practices and evaluating adherence to chronic pain guidelines in outpatient practices in the United States. J Pain 2013;14(6):568–78.

11. Gammons V, Caswell G. Older people and barriers to self-reporting of chronic pain. Br J Nurs 2014;23(5):274–8.

12. Purser L, Warfield K, Richardson C. Making pain visible: an audit and review of documentation to improve the use of pain assessment by implementing pain as the fifth vital sign. Pain Manag Nurs 2014;15(1):137–42.

13. Hwang U, Belland LK, Handel DA, et al. Is all pain treated equally? A multicenter evaluation of acute pain care by age. Pain 2014;155(12):2568–74.

14. Shega J, Dale W, Andrew M, et al. Persistent pain and frailty: a case for homeostenosis. J Am Geriatr Soc 2012;60:113–7.

15. Booker SS, Bartoszczyk DA, Herr KA. Pain management in frail elders. Am Nurse Today 2016;11(4):1–9.

16. Hadjistavropoulos T, Herr K, Prkachin KM, et al. Pain assessment in elderly adults with dementia. Lancet Neurol 2014;13(12):1216–27.

17. Ngu SSC, Tan MP, Subramanian P, et al. Pain assessment using self-reported, nurse-reported, and observational pain assessment tools among older individuals with cognitive impairment. Pain Manag Nurs 2015;16(4):595–601.

18. Herr K. Pain assessment strategies in older patients. J Pain 2011;12(3 Suppl 1): S3–13.

19. Chen YH, Lin LC. The credibility of self-reported pain among institutional older people with different degrees of cognitive function in Taiwan. Pain Manag Nurs 2015;16(3):163–72.

20. Lukas A, Niederecker T, Gunther I, et al. Self- and proxy report for the assessment of pain in patients with and without cognitive impairment: experiences gained in a geriatric hospital. Z Gerontol Geriatr 2013;46:214–21.

21. Buffum MD, Miaskowski C, Sands L, et al. A pilot study of the relationship between discomfort and agitation in patients with dementia. Geriatr Nurs 2001; 22(2):80–5.

22. Herr KA, Booker SS. Assessment of pain in persons with dementia. In: Lussier D, Cruciani RA, editors. Handbook of pain management in older persons. New York: Springer Publishing Company, in press.

23. Texas Department of Disability and Aging Services. Pain scale determination process. 2011. Available at: http://www.dads.state.tx.us/providers/qmp/docs/painscaledeterminationprocess.pdf. Accessed October 11, 2015.

24. Herr KA, Coyne PJ, McCaffery M, et al. Pain assessment in the patient unable to self-report: position statement with clinical practice recommendations. Pain Manag Nurs 2011;12(4):230–50.

25. Kovach CR, Noonan PE, Griffie J, et al. The assessment of discomfort in dementia protocol. Pain Manag Nurs 2002;3(1):16–27.

26. van Herk R, van Dijk M, Biemold N, et al. Assessment of pain: can caregivers or relatives rate pain in nursing home residents? J Clin Nurs 2009;18:2478–85.

27. Hadjistavropoulos T, Fitzgerald TD, Marchildon GP. Practice guidelines for assessing pain in older persons with dementia residing in long-term care facilities. Physiother Can 2010;62:104–13.

28. Salaffi F, Ciapetti A, Carotti M. Pain assessment strategies in patients with musculoskeletal conditions. Reumatismo 2012;64(4):216–29.

29. Hehl J, McDonald DD. Older adults' pain communication during ambulatory medical visits: an exploration of communication accommodation theory. Pain Manag Nurs 2014;15(2):466–73.

30. Eliades A, Mesko PJ. Developing and testing the effectiveness of the Mesko-Eliades pain area locator tool to assess pain location in children. 26th Sigma Theta Tau International Research Congress 2015. Puerto Rico. July 23-27, 2015.

31. McDonald DD, Shea M, Fedo J, et al. Older adult pain communication and the brief pain inventory short form. Pain Manag Nurs 2008;9(4):154–9.

32. Lalloo C, Jibb LA, Rivera J, et al. "There's a pain app for that": review of patient-targeted smartphone applications for pain management. Clin J Pain 2015;31: 557–63.

33. de la Vega R, Miro J. mHealth: a strategic field without a solid scientific soul. A systematic review of pain-related apps. PLoS One 2014;9(7):e101312.

34. Herr K, Spratt KF, Garand L, et al. Evaluation of the Iowa pain thermometer and other selected pain intensity scales in younger and older adult cohorts using controlled clinical pain: a preliminary study. Pain Med 2007;8:585–600.

35. International Association for the Study of Pain. Faces Pain Scale- Revised. 2001. Available at: http://www.iasp-pain.org/Education/Content.aspx?ItemNumber= 1519. Accessed October 15, 2015.

36. Ware LJ, Herr KA, Booker SS, et al. Psychometric evaluation of the revised Iowa Pain Thermometer (IPT-r) in a sample of cognitively intact and impaired diverse older adults: a pilot study. Pain Manag Nurs 2015;16(4):475–82.

37. Edelen MO, Saliba D. Correspondence of verbal descriptor and numeric rating scales for pain intensity: an item response theory calibration. J Gerontol A Biol Sci Med Sci 2010;65(7):778–85.

38. Jones KR, Vojir CP, Hutt E, et al. Determining mild, moderate, and severe pain equivalency across pain-intensity tools in nursing home residents. J Rehabil Res Dev 2007;44(2):305–14.

39. Gloth FM 3rd, Scheve AA, Stober CV, et al. The functional pain scale: reliability, validity, and responsiveness in an elderly population. J Am Med Dir Assoc 2001;2(3):110–4.

40. Arnstein P. Pain assessment. In: Arnstein P, editor. Clinical coach for effective pain management. Philadelphia: FA Davis Company; 2010. p. 63, 66.

41. Keller S, Bann CM, Dodd SL, et al. Validity of the brief pain inventory for use in documenting the outcomes of patients with non-cancer pain. Clin J Pain 2004; 20(5):309–18.

42. Blozik E, Stuck AE, Niemann S, et al. Geriatric pain measure short form: development and initial evaluation. J Am Geriatr Soc 2007;55(1):2045–50.

43. de Waal MWM, den Elzen WPJ, Achterberg WP, et al. A postal screener for pain and need for treatment in older persons in primary care. J Am Geriatr Soc 2014; 62:1832–7.

44. Stubbs B, Eggermont L, Patchay S, et al. Older adults with chronic musculoskeletal pain are at increased risk of recurrent falls and the brief pain inventory could help identify those most at risk. Geriatr Gerontol Int 2015;15(7):881–8.
45. Simmons SF, Schnelle JF, Saraf AA, et al. Pain and satisfaction with pain management among older patients during transition from acute to skilled nursing care. Gerontologist 2015. [Epub ahead of print].
46. Booker S, Haedtke C. Evaluating pain management in older adults. Nursing 2016; 46(6):66–9.
47. van Soest-Poortvliet MC, van der Steen JT, de Vet HCW, et al. Comfort goal of care and end-of-life outcomes in dementia: a prospective study. Palliat Med 2015;29(6):538–46.
48. Hwang U, Platts-Mills TF. Acute pain management in older adults in the emergency department. Clin Geriatr Med 2013;29:151–64.

# Interdisciplinary Approaches to Managing Pain in Older Adults

Abigail Wickson-Griffiths, RN, PhD[a],*,
Sharon Kaasalainen, RN, PhD[b], Keela Herr, RN, PhD[c]

## KEYWORDS

- Interdisciplinary • Multidisciplinary • Pain management • Older adults

## KEY POINTS

- An interdisciplinary approach to managing pain has been widely used in managing specific pain conditions (eg, lower back and fibromyalgia) but not reviewed specifically for older adults.
- Interdisciplinary approaches have been used in primary, residential long-term, and acute care settings, where a variety of health care professionals work on pain teams to manage pain in older adults.
- Given the multidimensional nature of pain in older adults, interdisciplinary approaches to managing pain are recommended in practice.

## INTRODUCTION

Worldwide, the population is aging,[1] and the onus is on health and other wellness care professionals to recognize issues that are common in older adults and strategize to meet their needs. In this context of aging, attention to pain management in later life is essential because untreated or undertreated pain has been consistently documented among both community-dwelling and facility-based dwelling older adults.[2] Although the prevalence of pain can vary by residential setting, chronic (or persistent) pain is experienced by 25% to 76% of older adults living in the community and between 83% and 93% of those residing in facility-based care.[3] Discovering and implementing effective strategies for aiding older adults in managing their pain is important because persistent pain can lead to a poor quality of life, including mental distress,

Disclosure Statement: Authors have nothing to disclose.
[a] Faculty of Nursing, University of Regina, 3737 Wascana Parkway, Regina, Saskatchewan S4S 0A2, Canada; [b] School of Nursing, McMaster University, 1280 Main Street West, HSC 3N25F, Hamilton, Ontario L8S 4K1, Canada; [c] College of Nursing, University of Iowa, 101 College of Nursing Building, 50 Newton Road, Iowa City, IA 52242-1121, USA
* Corresponding author.
*E-mail address:* Abigail.Wickson-Griffiths@uregina.ca

social isolation, and decreased cognitive and physical performance.[2,4] Certainly, persistent pain has been linked to disability and morbidity, which has a negative impact on the older adult. Given the multidimensional nature of pain,[5] however, an interdisciplinary or multidisciplinary (hereafter referred to as interdisciplinary) approach to its management in the older adult has been strongly encouraged (eg, American Geriatrics Society guidelines).[6–8] Interdisciplinary teams are typically made up of a variety of health and wellness care practitioners who work together to share their discipline-specific knowledge and skills to facilitate patient care.[9] This article reviews the rationale for an interdisciplinary approach for managing pain in older adults as well as studies that have used this approach.

## WHY THE NEED FOR AN INTERDISCIPLINARY APPROACH?
### Description of Pain in the Older Adult

Pain can be described as a multidimensional phenomenon, caused by noxious sensory stimuli or neuropathologic means, which cannot be separated from an individual's emotional response to it.[6] There is general consensus that the biopsychosocial model should guide how practitioners approach pain, that is, as an "interactive, psychophysiological behavior pattern" where the physical and psychosocial components cannot be teased apart or considered separately.[2] Within this understanding, practitioners acknowledge that older adults can and often do experience different types of pain, including persistent (ie, chronic), acute, cancer, and operative.[4,10] Due to the complexity of pain in the older adult, it is managed with different approaches as detailed in evidence-based guidelines (eg, "Practice Guidelines for Acute Pain Management in the Perioperative Setting,"[11] "Persistent Pain in Older Adults: Evidence-based Practice Guideline,"[12] and "Acute Pain Management in Older Adults: Evidence-based Practice Guideline"[13]). Given the physiologic, emotional, and social aspects of pain that are managed with different approaches depending on pain type, both medical (eg, physician, geriatrician, and anesthesiologist) and nonmedical (eg, social worker, dietitian, and pharmacist)[14] practitioners contribute to the older adult's overall well-being.

### Difficult Pain Management in the Older Adult

Overall, managing pain in older adults is frequently difficult due to physiologic changes and various psychosocial aspects that are age related, along with lack of knowledge on the part of many health care providers. Kress and colleagues[2] along with other investigators[5,15] have summarized key complications that should be considered in the older adult and which support the need for an interdisciplinary approach in the evaluation and follow-up of pain:

- A decrease in organ function (eg, liver and kidney filtration rates) and other physiologic changes (eg, fat/muscle composition), which can increase the chances of adverse side effects from pharmacologic agents
- An increase in the prevalence of comorbidities, which has a negative impact on overall health and complicates diagnosis of pain pathology
- The need for multiple medications to manage comorbidities, which can lead to polypharmacy
- Atypical (eg, sleep disturbances or agitation) or addition of acute pain symptoms in persistent pain conditions (eg, fracture in presence of arthritis)
- Poor reporting of pain among older adults with cognitive impairment, which may limit the ability to express pain; the misconception that pain is an expected part of aging; and older adults' fear of diagnostic tests and new diagnoses

- Poor management of pain on the part of the medical and nonmedical practitioners due to the belief that pain is an expected part of aging or that there is a reduced sensation of pain not requiring attention
- Poor knowledge of health care practitioners around appropriate pain management (eg, types/presentation of pain, assessment, treatment, and application of evidence-informed care)

These complications may be better addressed by a team of interdisciplinary professionals that can intervene on each according to their discipline-specific knowledge. In addition, a lack of knowledge about pain management may be positively influenced by working with knowledgeable colleagues. Core competencies for interprofessional prelicensure education have been published that help establish the importance of addressing pain using this approach.[16] Core competencies have been recommended in the following 4 domains:

- Multidimensional nature of pain
- Pain assessment and measurement
- Management of pain
- Context of pain management[16]

## A Comprehensive Approach is Recommended

In 2007, an "Interdisciplinary Expert Consensus Statement on Assessment of Pain in Older Adults"[7] was published that outlined 3 main domains for a comprehensive assessment (Fig. 1 in the original publication for schematic). A review of the 3 domains of assessment helps demonstrate the need for an interdisciplinary approach to pain management, including evaluation and follow-up in older adults. The 3 domains include

1. Initial determination and/or ongoing monitoring of pain. The initial determination of pain includes the older adult's self-report of pain, using both unidimensional (eg, pain thermometer scale[17]) and multidimensional (eg, Brief Pain Inventory[18]) measures and behavioral observations of pain (eg, Pain Assessment Checklist for Seniors with Limited Ability to Communicate-II,[19] Pain Assessment in Advanced Dementia,[20] and Abbey Pain Scale[21]) when appropriate.[7]
2. Medical, pharmacologic, and functional assessments of pain-related concerns. In this domain, a physical examination of the older adult includes assessments for pain during physical examination, functional and sensory impairments, age-specific physical concerns, pharmacology, and inflammation.[7]
3. Assessment of psychosocial factors contributing to the pain complaint. In this domain professionals should assess for psychosocial comorbidities and other factors that can moderate treatment outcomes, including psychological well-being, affective and interpersonal processes, cognitive processes (general and pain specific), pain-related disability (general and pain specific), personality, and coping.[7]

The following section presents the individual roles that may be involved in the interdisciplinary assessment and management of pain.

## Interdisciplinary Team and Roles in Pain Management

The need for the interdisciplinary team in helping to manage pain in older adults stems from the nature of pain as well as common complexity in its presentation in later life. Therefore, an interdisciplinary approach to managing pain from comprehensive assessment (discussed previously), pharmacotherapy, psychological support, physical rehabilitation and maintenance, and interventional procedures aspects is strongly recommended.[2,4] The interdisciplinary team offers the older adult both pharmacologic and nonpharmacologic treatments, consistent with the respective discipline's contributions. The literature shows that a variety of health and social/recreation practitioners work in multidisciplinary pain teams, although they are not necessarily dedicated to managing pain in older adults. For example, a study by Peng and colleagues[14] outlined a variety of medical and nonmedical practitioners working either full time or part time in multidisciplinary pain clinics across Canada to address the complex needs of patients in pain (**Box 1**). These teams are typically led, however, by anesthetists, psychologists or psychiatrists, and physiotherapists.[22] In an effort to encourage innovation in meeting the pain management needs of older adults, investigators have explored the emerging roles of the nurse practitioner[23] and occupational therapist within the interdisciplinary team.[24]

Each professional should work to the full scope of practice, contributing discipline-specific pain management knowledge and skills, while working collaboratively with colleagues. In an ideal selection of key members on an interdisciplinary team, it is

---

**Box 1**
**Examples of professionals working in multidisciplinary pain clinics**

*Medical*

Addiction specialist

Anesthesiologist

Family physician

Gynecologist

Internist

Neurologist

Neurosurgeon

Orthopedic surgeon

Psychiatrist

Rheumatologist


*Non medical*

Acupuncturist

Dentist

Dietitian

Kinesiologist

Nurse

Occupational therapist

Physiotherapist

Psychologist

Sex therapist

Social worker

*Data from* Peng P, Stinson JN, Choiniere M, et al. Role of health care professionals in multidisciplinary pain treatment facilities in Canada. Pain Res Manag 2008;13:484–8.

important to consider the pain problem addressed; in older adults, it is likely to be chronic or complex issues.[2] For example, the key members of a team addressing pain issues related to end-of-life care (eg, team of a primary care provider, nurse, and social worker) likely differ from those caring for an older adult in a restorative care program postfracture (eg, team of a primary care provider and physical and occupational therapists). An example of how different professionals may work together is provided by the Western Australian Department of Health[25] as follows:

- Generalist: leads the integration of pain treatment
- Physiotherapist: coordinates exercise and physical function activities
- Occupational therapist: manages employment (when appropriate) and recreational activities
- Clinical psychologist: manages emotional response to pain
- Dietitian: provide manages nutritional/meal plan guidance to reduce weight

No matter the composition of the interdisciplinary team, the older adult and a family caregiver should be central to a patient-centered team.[16] Ideally, they are an integral part of the interdisciplinary team's assessment, development of a plan, and decision making to ensure that management strategies match preferences and values and can be reasonably and consistently used by the older adult.[26] It follows that although the composition of the team may differ depending on local resource availability, increasing access to technology, such as telemedicine[27] and other secure Web-based applications, can help to connect older adults with specialist or relevant disciplines to help support their pain care. Overall, the older adult's access to multiple disciplines may help to better meet their individual needs (eg, social support, management of polypharmacy, psychological support, and routine nursing monitoring/assessment) and ensure quality pain management outcomes.[28]

### Challenges of Assembling and Working in Interdisciplinary Teams

Although an interdisciplinary approach to managing older adult care, including pain in later life, is routinely encouraged,[7,29] general challenges and barriers to implementing this type of care have been documented at the system, team, and individual levels.[30] Examples include

- System level
  - Lack of reimbursement for multiple providers[30]
  - Nondrug therapies not covered or limited by insurers (eg, massage therapy)[31]
- Team/individual level
  - Lack of knowledge around scope of practice and competencies of other disciplines[26]
  - Power imbalances or turf wars[26]
  - Distrust among collaborating team members[26,32]

At the system level, reimbursement for multiple providers warrants ongoing consideration, despite best practices for pain care highlighting the importance of interdisciplinary care teams, particularly to address chronic pain problems. Exemplars exist in the environment of hospice and palliative care teams; however, these services are limited to those either at the end of life or those with advanced life-threatening illness.[33] Current reimbursement structures in the United States provide financial reimbursement through Medicare for hospice interdisciplinary team services,[33] but a mechanism for reimbursing interdisciplinary team contributions to the pain treatment plan has not been available.[34] With the advent of the Patient Protection Affordable

Care Act, emphasis on person-centered care and medical homes, in which interdisciplinary assessment and treatment activities are coordinated, may provide a future avenue for support.[35] Moving from a fee-for-service structure to a fee-for–managing a patient's medical condition(s) has also promoted scrutiny of the treatment plan to assure access, quality care, and cost-effective patient outcomes,[36] perhaps highlighting the potential benefit of interdisciplinary collaboration.

### Summary of Evidence that Interdisciplinary Pain Care Teams Are Effective

Aside from the support to include interdisciplinary approaches in pain management, in general, practice-based interprofessional care results in improved care processes as well as outcomes for patients.[37] Given the support of interdisciplinary team management for pain, health care and other wellness practitioners have met the challenge to provide this type of team-based care. Systematic reviews of the outcomes of interdisciplinary care for chronic pain[38] and lower back pain[39] reveal moderate evidence to support the efficacy of multidisciplinary care. As recognized by Kirksey and colleagues,[40] however, the specific interdisciplinary approaches for older adults have not yet been reviewed.

Interdisciplinary approaches to managing pain in older adults have been evaluated in both the residential long-term care and acute care settings.[41–46] In all cases, interdisciplinary pain teams (with at least 2 disciplines) or work groups have been assembled to implement practices to alleviate or improve pain management among older adults, with or without cognitive impairment. For the most part, these approaches were based mainly on the implementation of guidelines (eg, from American Geriatric Society, American Medical Directors Association, and University of Iowa, College of Nursing, Hartford Center of Geriatric Nursing Excellence). The composition of each team varied (**Table 1**); however, nurses and physicians/medical professionals were commonly represented in all approaches. In addition to managing pain among older adults (and family members where applicable), individuals on the interdisciplinary teams could also act as a "go to" for other frontline staff, providing point-of-care education or more formal education on pain management to their peers. Overall, it is apparent that interdisciplinary approaches to care vary in terms of professional composition across settings as well as intended outcomes of the evaluated approaches. Given funding limitations, it is important to determine which interdisciplinary colleagues are essential given the unique circumstances of each older person's pain problem and care circumstances. It is encouraging that interdisciplinary teams are informing their practice on existing guidelines aimed at managing pain in the older adults.

In addition to the studies included in **Table 1**, many older adults receive pain care and other health care in the primary care setting. Commonly, patients in the United States depend on primary care for their management of pain.[47] In this setting it is important to have access to the interdisciplinary expertise needed to manage complex pain problems in this population. Interdisciplinary approaches to pain care have been evaluated and processes documented in the primary care setting, although perhaps not always specific to the older adult. Two examples include the Study of the Effectiveness of a Collaborative Approach to Pain[48] and the Stepped Care to Optimize Pain Care Effectiveness.[49] Both of these well-designed and conducted randomized controlled trials demonstrated the effectiveness of an interdisciplinary approach of managing pain in the primary care setting. Dobscha and colleagues[48] found modest improvement in pain-related disability, pain intensity, and depression in patients with baseline depression when a psychologist care manager and internist collaboratively assisted the patient and primary care provider (ie, either physician, physician

**Table 1**
Study summary

| Study, Location, Setting | Study Design | Interdisciplinary Pain Team Members | Interdisciplinary Pain Approach | Primary Findings |
|---|---|---|---|---|
| Kaasalainen et al,[41] 2012, Canada, Long-term care | Controlled pre–post; long-term care home control site | Administrators, family physicians, advanced practice nurses, pharmacists, licensed nurses (registered nurses, registered practical nurses), personal support workers, social workers, and physiotherapist<br>• Met most consistently during intervention | To implement a pain protocol (AMDA/AGS-based); IP team was developed, pain education and skills training<br>Monthly meetings with IP team review<br>• Resident pain issues<br>• Coordinate and provide formal education to other staff<br>• Provide informal/point of care education | Less pain after 1 y for residents living in long-term care home with IP team; increased use of assessment tools and pain documentation; IP team helped to successfully implement protocol |
| Kelly,[42] 2008, USA, Long-term care | Descriptive | Social worker, pastoral care counselor, rehabilitation therapist, therapeutic activity worker<br>• IP team collaborated with physician and family members<br>• Nurses were responsible to ensure plan of care was implemented | Upon admission to long-term care, nursing assessed pain for 7 d, including a comprehensive assessment if pain present; referral to IP program if pain present<br>Weekly meetings with IP team to individualize treatment plans for residents in collaboration with physician and family<br>IP team responsible for providing education and presentations (education cart and bulletin board) | Reports of increased competency and reputation for pain management, increased referral from physicians to IP program, requested to provide IP education to other facilities, improved resident function |

*(continued on next page)*

**Table 1**
*(continued)*

| Study, Location, Setting | Study Design | Interdisciplinary Pain Team Members | Interdisciplinary Pain Approach | Primary Findings |
|---|---|---|---|---|
| Laguna et al,[43] 2012, USA, Acute/critical care hospital | Pre–post | Palliative care physicians (n = 2), social worker, nurse<br>• Hospital chaplain as needed | Palliative care physicians and nurse trained on procedures<br>IP team provided patients with consultation about physical, psychological, social and spiritual needs for end-of-life care;<br>IP team addressed pain and symptom control needs and established patient discharge plans | Pain decreased after IP team consultation and throughout hospital stay; however, pain increased 10 d post discharge from hospital |
| McLeish et al,[44] 2009, Australia, Acute care hospital | Quality-improvement initiative | Nurses, nurse pain specialists, geriatrician, pharmacist, physiotherapist, clinical psychologist | 4 phases of interdisciplinary team work to improve pain practice:<br>1. Describing and identifying clinical issue (pain), and reviewing appropriate practice standards<br>2. Measuring pain management activity<br>3. Taking action to improve pain management practice<br>4. Reviewing and sharing findings | IP team found gaps in assessing and managing pain in older adults without verbal communication abilities; staff did not routinely document specific pain assessments, Abbey Pain Scale was implemented |

| Philips et al,[45] 2005, USA, Long-term care | Descriptive | Physicians, pharmacists, nurses, physical and occupational therapists, speech pathologists, social workers, dietitians, nursing assistants, and administrators | IP team focused on enhancing residents' well-being and implemented acute/chronic pain treatment program based on AMDA and AGS guidelines and recommendations. IP team developed an educational program and trained frontline staff to assess and manage pain Weekly meetings held with the interdisciplinary team to review each resident's plan of care and shared with other team members | None reported |
| Titler et al,[46] 2009, USA, Acute care hospitals | Experimental | Nurses, physicians | A TRIP model was used to implement the acute pain management in the elderly guideline with nurses and physicians managing older adults' hip fractures Along with success of implementation, pain intensity was measured | Patients with hip fractures receiving the TRIP approach to implementation of the guideline (vs usual care) had lower pain intensity |

*Abbreviations:* AGS, American Geriatrics Society; AMDA, American Medical Directors Association; IP, interdisciplinary pain; TRIP, translating research into practice.
*Data from* Refs.[41–46]

assistant, or nurse practitioner). In addition, Kroenke and colleagues[49] demonstrated the effectiveness of an intervention by a nurse case manager and a physician pain specialist collaboratively assisting a patient's primary care physician in managing chronic musculoskeletal pain. Patients receiving the collaborative care had significantly improved pain intensity and were more likely to have positive reports of global pain improvement, pain medication prescriptions, and overall pain treatment than the care as usual counterparts at 12 months.

## SUMMARY

An interdisciplinary approach to managing pain in the older adult, regardless of care setting, is encouraged in the evidence-based literature and practice guidelines. Despite some of the noted barriers and challenges to implementing an interdisciplinary approach, given the multidimensional nature of pain, a variety of health care professionals (both medical and nonmedical) can contribute their expertise in a collaborative manner to assist in its successful management among older adults. The literature provides examples of different interdisciplinary team compositions, which may depend on resource availability; however, the patient and family should always be included in the team. Overall, an interdisciplinary approach to pain management is strongly recommended in this population.

## REFERENCES

1. United Nations. Department of Economic and Social Affairs, Population Division. World population ageing 2013. 2013. Available at: http://www.un.org/en/development/desa/population/publications/pdf/ageing/WorldPopulationAgeing2013.pdf. Accessed December 1, 2015.
2. Kress HG, Ahlbeck K, Aldington D, et al. Managing chronic pain in elderly patients requires a CHANGE of approach. Curr Med Res Opin 2014;30:1154–63.
3. Abdulla A, Adams N, Bone M, et al. Guidance on the management of pain in older people. Age Ageing 2013;42:i1–57.
4. Cavalieri TA. Management of pain in older adults. J Am Osteopath Assoc 2005;105:S12–7.
5. Yonan CA, Wegener ST. Assessment and management of pain in the older adult. Rehabil Psychol 2003;48:4–13.
6. AGS Panel on Persistent Pain in Older Persons. The management of persistent pain in older Persons. J Am Geriatr Soc 2002;50:205–24.
7. Hadjistavropoulos T, Herr K, Turk DC, et al. An interdisciplinary expert consensus statement on assessment of pain in older adults. Clin J Pain 2007;2:S1–43.
8. Pergolizzi J, Ahlbeck K, Aldington D, et al. The development of chronic pain: physiological CHANGE necessitates a multidisciplinary approach to treatment. Curr Med Res Opin 2013;29:1127–35.
9. Nancarrow SA, Booth A, Ariss S, et al. Ten principles of good interdisciplinary team work. Hum Resour Health 2013;11:19.
10. Urban D, Cherny N, Catane R. The management of cancer pain in the elderly. Crit Rev Oncol Hematol 2010;73:176–83.
11. American Society of Anesthesiologists Task Force on Acute Pain Management. Practice guidelines for acute pain management in the perioperative setting. Anesthesiology 2012;116:248–73.
12. Arnstein PA, Herr K. Persistent pain in older adults. Evidence-based practice guideline. Iowa City (IA): The University of Iowa; Hartford Center of Geriatric Nursing Excellence; 2015.

13. Cornelius R, Herr K, Gordon D, et al. Acute pain management in older adults. Evidence-practice guideline. Iowa City (IA): The University of Iowa; Csomay Center of Gerontological Excellence; 2016.
14. Peng P, Stinson JN, Choiniere M, et al. Role of health care professionals in multidisciplinary pain treatment facilities in Canada. Pain Res Manag 2008;13:484–8.
15. Planton J, Edlund B. Regulatory components for treating persistent pain in long-term care. J Gerontol Nurs 2010;36:49–56.
16. Fishman S, Young HM, Arwood EL. Core competencies for pain management: results of an interprofessional consensus summit. Pain Med 2013;14:971–81.
17. Herr K, Spratt KF, Garand L, et al. Evaluation of the Iowa pain thermometer and other selected pain intensity scales in younger and older adult cohorts using controlled clinical pain: a preliminary study. Pain Med 2007;8:585–600.
18. Cleeland CS, Ryan KM. Pain assessment: global use of the brief pain inventory. Ann Acad Med Singapore 1994;23:129–38.
19. Chan S, Hadjistavropolous T, Williams J, et al. Evidenced-based development and initial validation of the pain assessment checklist for seniors with limited ability to communicate-II (PACSLAC-II). Clin J Pain 2014;30:816–24.
20. Warden V, Hurley AC, Volicer L. Development and psychometric evaluation of the pain assessment in advanced dementia (PAINAD) scale. J Am Med Dir Assoc 2003;4:9–15.
21. Abbey J, Piller N, De Bellis A. The Abbey pain scale: a 1-minute numerical indicator for people with end-stage dementia. Int J Palliat Nurs 2004;10:6–13.
22. Corran T, Helme RD, Gibson ST. Multidisciplinary assessment and treatment of pain in older persons. Top Geriatr Rehabil 2001;16:1–11.
23. Kaasalainen S, Martin-Misener R, Carter N, et al. The nurse practitioner role in pain management in long-term care. J Adv Nurs 2010;66:542–51.
24. Zimmerman B. The occupational therapist's role in the management of persistent pain in older adults. WFOT BULL 2003;48:13–35.
25. Government of Western Australia. Department of Health. Pain management team. 2013. Available at: http://painhealth.csse.uwa.edu.au/resources/painHEALTH-using-a-pain-team.pdf. Accessed December 1, 2015.
26. Orchard CA, Curran V, Kabene S. Creating a culture for interdisciplinary collaborative professional practice. Med Educ Online 2005;10:11.
27. Ontario Telemedicine Network. 2015. Available at: https://otn.ca/en. Accessed February 14, 2016.
28. American Pain Society. Interdisciplinary pain management. Available at: http://americanpainsociety.org/uploads/about/position-statements/interdisciplinary-white-paper.pdf. Accessed December 1, 2015.
29. Partnership for Health in Aging Workgroup on Interdisciplinary Team Training in Geriatrics. Position statement on interdisciplinary team training in geriatrics: an essential component of quality health care for older adults. J Am Geriatr Soc 2014;62:961–5.
30. Grant RW, Finnocchio LJ, California Primary Care Consortium Subcommittee on Interdisciplinary Collaboration. Interdisciplinary collaborative teams in primary care: a model curriculum and resource guide. San Francisco (CA): Pew Health Professions Commission; 1995.
31. Frass M, Strassl RP, Friehs H. Use and acceptance of complementary and alternative medicine among the general population and medical personnel: a systematic review. Ochsner J 2012;12:45–56.
32. Kaasalainen S, Coker E, Dolovich L, et al. Pain management decision making among long-term care physicians and nurses. West J Nurs Res 2007;29:561–80.

33. Meier D. Increased access to palliative care and hospice services: opportunities to improve value in health care. Milbank Q 2011;89:343–80.

34. American Geriatrics Society Expert Panel on Person-Centered Care. Person-centered care: a definition and essential elements. J Am Geriatr Soc 2016;64:15–8.

35. Kogan AC, Wilber K, Mosqueda L. Person-centered care for older adults with chronic conditions and functional impairment: a systematic literature review. J Am Geriatr Soc 2016;64:e1–7.

36. Westphal EC, Alkema G, Seidel R, et al. How to get better care with lower costs? see the person, not the patient. J Am Geriatr Soc 2016;64:19–21.

37. Zwarenstein M, Reeves S, Goldman J. Interprofessional collaboration: effects of practice-based interventions on professional practice and healthcare outcomes. Cochrane Database Syst Rev 2009;(8):CD000072.

38. Scascighini L, Toma V, Dober-Spielmann S. Multidisciplinary treatment for chronic pain: a systematic review of interventions and outcomes. Rheumatology 2008;47:670–8.

39. Kamper SJ, Apeldoorn AT, Chiarotto A. Multidisciplinary biopsychosocial rehabilitation for chronic low back pain: cochrane systematic review and meta-analysis. BMJ 2015;350:h444.

40. Kirksey KM, McGlory G, Sefcik EF. Pain assessment and management in critically ill older adults. Crit Care Nurs Q 2015;38:237–44.

41. Kaasalainen S, Brazil K, Akhtar-Danesh N, et al. The evaluation of an interdisciplinary pain protocol in long term care. J Am Med Dir Assoc 2012;664:e1–8.

42. Kelly AM. Making pain management a priority: managing suffering for the elderly takes multi-faceted approach. Health Prog 2008;89:62–4.

43. Laguna J, Goldstein R, Allen J, et al. Inpatient palliative care and patient pain: pre-and post-outcomes. J Pain Symptom Manage 2012;43:1051–9.

44. McLeish P, Mungall D, Wiechula R. Are we providing the best possible pain management for our elderly patients in the acute-care setting? Int J Evid Based Healthc 2009;7:173–80.

45. Philips SL, Southworth A, Myers M, et al. Pain management in a long-term care setting: an interdisciplinary approach. Ann Longterm Care 2005;13:1.

46. Titler MG, Herr K, Brooks JM, et al. Translating research into practice intervention improves management of acute pain in older hip fracture patients. Health Serv Res 2009;44:264–87.

47. McCarberg BH. Pain management in primary care: strategies to mitigate opioid misuse, abuse, and diversion. Postgrad Med 2011;123:119–30.

48. Dobscha SK, Corson K, Perrin NA, et al. Collaborative care for chronic pain in primary care: a cluster randomized trial. JAMA 2009;301:1242–52.

49. Kroenke K, Krebs EE, Wu J, et al. Telecare collaborative management of chronic pain in primary care: a randomized clinical trial. JAMA 2014;312:240–8.

# Pharmacotherapies in Geriatric Chronic Pain Management

Zachary A. Marcum, PharmD, PhD[a], Nakia A. Duncan, PharmD[b], Una E. Makris, MD, MSc[c],*

## KEYWORDS

- Chronic pain • Medication • Older adults • Adverse drug events • Polypharmacy

## KEY POINTS

- Pharmacologic management for chronic pain is one part of the multimodal, interdisciplinary approach to the treatment of chronic pain in older adults.
- Topical agents are ideal for an older adult with localized pain that is uncontrolled with other medications (or if specific classes of medications are contraindicated).
- Use of the lowest effective dose of all pharmacologic agents, and consideration of low-dose combination therapy, are especially appropriate in older adults with chronic pain.
- Engage the older adult in determining patient-centered treatment goals and expectations of pain management.
- Establish a careful surveillance plan to determine whether treatment goals are being met and for monitoring potential toxicity of pharmacotherapies for chronic pain.

Pain is highly prevalent, costly, and frequently disabling in later life.[1–6] It is most often owing to musculoskeletal causes,[7] usually involves multiple sites,[8] and rarely occurs in the absence of other comorbidities.[9] Consistent with other geriatric syndromes, chronic pain in older adults often develops via a multifactorial pathway, resulting in various sequelae including poor self-reported health and quality of life, disability, impaired ambulation, depression, and decreased socialization, as well as falls, low energy, and impaired sleep.[6,10–13]

Disclosure Statement: Dr Z.A. Marcum is a consultant for Purdue Pharma. Drs N.A. Duncan and U.E. Makris have nothing to disclose.
Funded by: National Institutes of Health Grant number(s): KL2TR001103; UL1TR001105.
[a] Department of Pharmacy, University of Washington School of Pharmacy, 1959 Northeast Pacific Avenue, Box 357630, Seattle, WA 98195, USA; [b] Texas Tech University Health Sciences Center School of Pharmacy, 4500 South Lancaster Street, Building 7, Room 215, Dallas, TX, USA; [c] Division of Rheumatic Diseases, Department of Internal Medicine, VA North Texas Health Care System, UT Southwestern Medical Center, 5323 Harry Hines Boulevard, Dallas, TX 75390-9169, USA
* Corresponding author.
E-mail address: una.makris@utsouthwestern.edu

## CHALLENGES TO MANAGING PAIN IN LATER LIFE

Barriers to managing chronic pain effectively in older populations[14] include a limited evidence base to guide management,[15] lack of health care professional education,[16] health care professionals' concerns about the potential for treatment-related harm,[17] and older adults' beliefs about pain and pain treatments.[18] Other barriers specific to geriatric populations include age-related physiologic changes resulting in altered drug absorption and decreased renal excretion, sensory impairments, polypharmacy, and multimorbidity.[15] There is limited evidence in the literature to guide pharmacologic management because older adults are often underrepresented or excluded from clinical trials.[15,19-21] More specifically, the presence of multiple comorbid conditions such as[22] cognitive impairment, gait disorders, and kidney, lung, and cardiovascular disease often serve as exclusion criteria in drug trials. Further, it is important to recognize that the pain experience, values, and priorities may be different among older adults as compared with younger adults,[23-25] and that it is not appropriate to use a "one size fits all" approach when applying guidelines from younger to older populations.

## EXISTING GUIDELINES FOR MANAGING CHRONIC PAIN IN LATER LIFE

Two guidelines and several consensus statements provide useful information regarding the assessment and management of chronic pain in older adults (Appendix 1 lists additional resources).[10,26-29] The American Geriatrics Society guideline (last updated in 2009) provides recommendations on the initiation and titration of commonly used pharmacotherapies.[28,29] Given the complexity of managing older adults with chronic pain, experts agree that these patients are most likely to benefit from an interdisciplinary team approach. This team may consist of various health care providers, including those in primary care, gerontology, geriatrics, rheumatology, physical medicine and rehabilitation, physical and occupational therapists, pharmacy, nursing services, social work, and psychiatry/psychology. There is agreement across guidelines about the need to intervene aggressively using an interdisciplinary approach that includes both pharmacologic and nonpharmacologic treatments. Pain relief is one of the most commonly endorsed goals of older adults.[30] To achieve this goal, collaborative care approaches have been found to be effective. One randomized controlled trial found that a collaborative multicomponent intervention that included physician and patient education, activation, and symptom monitoring in targeted primary care patients with chronic pain was associated with significant improvement in pain-related disability, pain intensity, and depressive symptom scores over a 12-month period.[31]

In 2016, the Centers for Disease Control and Prevention (CDC) released updated guidelines for opioid use in chronic pain. Overall, the guideline is intended to improve communication about benefits and risks of opioids for chronic pain, improve safety and effectiveness of pain treatment, and reduce risks associated with long-term opioid therapy. Of great importance, non-opioid therapy is emphasized as the preferred treatment for chronic pain.[32,33]

In this article, we provide a review of nonopioid pharmacotherapies for chronic pain management in older adults. The safety and efficacy of opioids for the treatment of noncancer pain is covered by Dr. Naples and colleagues (See, "The Role of Opioid Analgesics in Geriatric Pain Management," in this issue).

## Specific Pharmacologic Agents

### Topicals

Topical medications provide a unique pathway to control pain that is localized and less likely to be absorbed systemically.[34,35] This route of administration is particularly important for older adults who often take multiple medications, because it decreases the likelihood of side effects, drug–drug interactions, and overall pill burden.[35] However, skin integrity must be considered with all topical products. With age, the skin becomes less hydrated and the epidermal layer thins. Absorption of topical medications can be affected by decreased hydration, tissue thickness, and surface lipids on the skin. The decreased lipid layer makes it more difficult for transdermal medications (eg, lidocaine patches) to penetrate the skin, because they are designed for gradual absorption and rely on intact, well-hydrated skin with adequate circulation. Dry or thin skin without a good subcutaneous layer can inhibit absorption of the drug potentially leading to variable treatment effects.[34,35] In addition, owing to decreased blood flow, doses or frequency may need to be adjusted to compensate for drug reservoir formation.[35]

Available topical medications include menthol, capsaicin, lidocaine, and diclofenac; **Table 1** details the indications, dose ranges, formulations, and clinical pearls for topical analgesics.

### Menthol/Methyl Salicylate

Menthol is available in many creams and patches over the counter. It causes a cooling sensation along with pain relief via counterirritant effects.[36] Menthol products are ideal for older adults (often used as adjunctive therapy) to treat minor pains because they have minimal side effects.

### Capsaicin

Capsaicin is derived from hot peppers and is available over the counter as a cream or by prescription as a highly concentrated patch.[34,37] Over time, capsaicin application desensitizes epidermal nociceptive nerves and decreases substance P, leading to pain reduction.[34,38] If an individual can tolerate the burning sensation with application for 1 to 2 weeks, the burning usually subsides. Capsaicin has been studied in patients with postherpetic neuralgia (PHN), diabetic neuropathy, and osteoarthritis (OA).[39] The high-dose patch, Qutenza, has been studied in PHN with a pooled number needed to treat of 6 to 9 over 12 weeks of application (median age of participants across trials was 71 years).[40] Additionally, low-dose (0.025% to 0.075%) creams have consistently shown improvement in pain compared with placebo over 4 to 8 weeks of therapy for PHN, OA, and diabetic neuropathy.[41–43] In PHN, continued response for up to 12 months was documented in a study that originally followed patients for 8 weeks. After 8 weeks, 48% had pain relief. Of this group, pain relief continued for 72% of participants.[43]

### Lidocaine

Lidocaine is available in various cream formulations and as a patch. Lidocaine decreases pain by blocking sodium ion channels, thereby stopping afferent pain signals.[34] The American Geriatrics Society recommends topical lidocaine for neuropathic pain.[29] The lidocaine patch is applied for 12 hours and removed for 12 hours, making it a poor choice for a cognitively impaired individual managing his or her own medications.

**Table 1**
**Topical agents**

| Medication | Indication | Preparation Strength | Formulations | Clinical Pearls |
|---|---|---|---|---|
| Menthol and menthol salicylate (BenGay, Icy Hot, Salonpas Arthritis Pain) | Generalized pain, minor aches and pain of muscle and joints (arthritis, backache, sprains, strains) | Methyl salicylate 10% Menthol 1.5%–3% | Cream, foam, patch | • Do not leave patch on for >8 h (max 2 patches/24 h) <br>• Avoid applying to wounds or damaged skin <br>• Avoid concurrent use with other topical agents |
| Capsaicin (Zostrix, Salonpas Gel patch, Qutenza) | Generalized pain, osteoarthritis, postherpetic neuralgia, diabetic neuropathy, HIV neuropathy (off-label use) | 0.025%–8% | Cream, gel, lotion, patch | • Several products available over the counter <br>• Caution burns at application site, recommend applying with gloves <br>• High-dose patch (Qutenza) may cause transient increases in blood pressure (monitor) |
| Lidocaine (Lidoderm, Xylocaine) | Generalized pain, postherpetic neuralgia, topical anesthesia | 2%–5% | Cream, gel, jelly, lotion, ointment, oral solution, patch | Use lowest amount necessary for pain relief; a large amount of these products applied for prolonged periods of time increases systemic absorption potentially leading to increased central nervous system and cardiac effects |
| Diclofenac (Solaraze, Flector, Pennsaid, Voltaren) | Generalized pain, Osteoarthritis (evaluated for hand and knee osteoarthritis) | 1%–3% | Cream, gel, solution, patch | • Limited data in older adults with baseline renal insufficiency and taking anticoagulants; monitor carefully <br>• Apply per physician or drug package insert instructions |

*Abbreviation:* HIV, human immunodeficiency virus.

## Topical Diclofenac

Widely used for more than 30 years outside of the United States, topical diclofenac sodium was the first topical NSAID approved by the US Food and Drug Administration (FDA) in 2007. It is often used for knee or hand OA-related pain. The literature on topical NSAIDs for sports injuries, musculoskeletal pain, or inflammatory arthritis has focused on subjects younger than 65 years old.[44,45] Available data suggest that some topical NSAIDs have comparable, or somewhat lower, efficacy than oral NSAIDs.[46,47] Even if less effective, these agents may be a reasonable option because their safety profile is superior to that of oral NSAIDs.[48] A systematic review of the literature evaluated safety of topical NSAIDS in older adults (age >60 years old) and showed that topical NSAIDs are almost as effective and carry a lower risk of severe adverse effects (gastrointestinal [GI]) as compared with oral NSAIDs.[49] There are limited data in older adults with baseline renal impairment or who are anticoagulated to understand potential adverse events of topical NSAIDS in these populations. Patients should be counseled that topical NSAID users have reported non–life-threatening GI events and many application site adverse events; thus, they are not entirely without risk.

## General Considerations

With all topical medications, patients should be instructed to not apply the medication to open skin or apply heat to the area because this may increase systemic absorption. Topical agents are considered an ideal adjunct agent for an older adult with localized pain that is uncontrolled with other medications (or if specific classes of medications are contraindicated). Of note, care should be taken when disposing patches to avoid the unintentional consumption by children or pets (see **Table 1**).

## Acetaminophen

The analgesic activity of acetaminophen (APAP) results from the central inhibition of prostaglandin synthesis. Yet, the primary mechanism of prostaglandin synthesis inhibition by APAP remains unknown.[50] Several studies have investigated the pharmacokinetic properties of APAP in healthy older adults and have reported varying effects of age.[50] APAP is rapidly and completely absorbed from the GI tract, and neither the rate nor the extent of absorption seems to be age dependent.[50] The volume of distribution decreases with age and female sex, which is consistent with the drug's hydrophilic nature as well as age-associated changes in body composition; no differences have been reported in the volume of distribution between healthy and frail older adults.[50] In general, advanced age does not alter the clearance of APAP, which is metabolized by phase II hepatic conjugative metabolism. However, some studies suggest that the metabolism of APAP in older adults is greatly variable and that the intrinsic conjugative activity of the liver may be preserved in healthy older adults but may be compromised in the frail elderly. It is unknown whether these changes in pharmacokinetic properties are responsible for increases in APAP hepatotoxicity.

APAP is recommended as a first-line analgesic for mild-to-moderate pain owing to OA of the knee and hip in multiple guidelines.[50] However, mounting evidence of its limited effectiveness (compared with placebo and other analgesics) and growing safety concerns have shifted opinions in recent years.[51–54] For example, the comparative effectiveness of available treatments for knee OA were evaluated in a systematic review and network metaanalysis.[52] Included studies were randomized trials of adults with knee OA comparing 2 or more of the following: APAP, diclofenac, ibuprofen, naproxen, celecoxib, intraarticular (IA) corticosteroids, IA hyaluronic acid, oral placebo, and IA placebo. A total of 137 studies comprising 33,243 participants were included, and 3-month outcomes of pain, function, and stiffness were assessed as the primary outcomes. The median age of participants across trials was 62 years. For pain, all interventions were statistically significantly better than oral placebo, with effect sizes ranging from 0.18 for the least efficacious treatment (APAP) to 0.63 for the most efficacious treatment (IA hyaluronic acid). Moreover, all treatments except APAP met the prespecified criteria for a clinically significant improvement in pain. Compared with APAP, naproxen, ibuprofen, diclofenac, IA hyaluronic acid, and IA corticosteroids were significantly superior for pain control. However, celecoxib was not found to be significantly better than APAP. For function, naproxen, ibuprofen, diclofenac, and celecoxib were significantly better than APAP. In terms of safety, oral nonselective NSAIDs led to more GI adverse events and withdrawals owing to adverse events than oral placebo and APAP, whereas these events were similar between APAP and celecoxib.

Another study was conducted using a systematic review and metaanalysis of placebo-controlled randomized trials to examine the efficacy and safety of APAP in the management of low back pain and OA of the hip or knee.[53] Thirteen randomized trials were included, and the investigators reported that there was "high-quality" evidence (based on the GRADE criteria) that APAP is ineffective for reducing pain intensity and disability or improving quality of life in the short term in people with low back pain. For hip or knee OA, there was "high-quality" evidence that APAP has a significant, although not clinically important, effect on pain and disability in the short term. More specifically, APAP was found to have a small effect (ie, <4 points on a 0–100 point scale) on pain, which is not likely to be meaningful for patients or their clinicians. In addition, the number of patients reporting any adverse events was similar in the APAP and placebo groups. In summary, this study found APAP to be ineffective for the treatment of low back pain and to provide a minimal short-term benefit for people with OA. The authors suggested that these results should lead to a reconsideration of APAP being a first-line treatment in clinical practice guidelines for low back pain and hip or knee OA.

Finally, a systematic review assessed the adverse event profile of APAP in the general adult population.[54] Eight cohort studies were included, and the main outcomes examined were all-cause mortality, cardiovascular adverse drug events (incident myocardial infarction, cerebrovascular accident, and hypertension), GI bleeding, and renal (reductions in estimated glomerular filtration rate, increases in serum creatinine, and need for renal replacement therapy) events. Given the known limitations of observational data (eg, confounding by indication), the results demonstrated a consistent dose-response association between APAP at standard analgesic doses and adverse drug events that are often observed with NSAIDs. For example, this review reported a dose–response association between APAP and increasing incidence of mortality, cardiovascular, GI, and renal adverse drug events. Furthermore, given the risk of APAP overdose, new regulations went into effect in 2014 that decreased the amount of APAP allowed in prescription products from 500 to 325 mg.[55] These new regulations do not include over-the-counter products.

Whereas prior and current guidelines recommend APAP as first-line therapy for the treatment of OA in older adults, recent evidence of uncertain analgesic benefit and increased safety concerns suggest a shifting risk–benefit profile.[56] Until further evidence becomes available, clinicians should continue evaluating the risk versus benefit when prescribing APAP using patient-specific information. Known risk factors for APAP-related adverse drug events, such as a renal impairment, hepatic dysfunction, and alcohol abuse, should be considered, and adequate dosing trials should be attempted before discontinuing APAP. Because APAP is the most commonly used analgesic and is available over the counter, patient education is important to communicate the known risks and benefit[55] (**Table 2**).

### Nonsteroidal antiinflammatory drugs

NSAIDs are one of the most common classes of drugs used to treat chronic pain owing to OA and other musculoskeletal disorders in older adults.[57–59] Specifically, an estimated 40% of the population age 65 years and older fill one or more prescriptions for an NSAID each year.[60] Considering that NSAIDs are also currently available over the counter, it is assumed that an even greater number of older adults in the United States take NSAIDs in an effort to relieve their pain. Although these agents can be effective in treating inflammation and pain, older adults are at increased risk for adverse drug events owing to age-related loss of physiologic organ reserve, increased comorbidities, polypharmacy, and changes in pharmacokinetics.[29] As a result, NSAID use causes an estimated 41,000 hospitalizations and 3300 deaths each year among older adults.[58] Some specific adverse drug events of concern with chronic use of NSAIDs include GI, renal, cardiovascular, cerebrovascular, and central nervous system (CNS) adverse effects.[61]

Two of the most serious adverse drug events associated with NSAID use are serious GI bleeds and cardiovascular events, such as myocardial infraction and stroke.[62] In 2005, the FDA issued a warning that NSAID use could cause heart attacks and strokes that could lead to death.[62] To help minimize these risks, the FDA also issued a public health advisory stating that "NSAIDs should be administered at the lowest effective dose for the shortest duration consistent with individual patient treatment goals."[63] Moreover, in 2015 the FDA strengthened this warning, based on a comprehensive review of new safety information, stating that all prescription NSAID labels need to

**Table 2**
**Acetaminophen**

| Medication | Indication | Dosage Range | Clinical Pearls |
|---|---|---|---|
| Acetaminophen (APAP; Tylenol) | Mild-to-moderate pain | Starting dose for older adults is same as for younger adults<br>Consider dose reduction in older adults with risk factors for acetaminophen-related toxicities, for example, frailty, alcohol use ($\geq$3 drinks per day), existing liver insufficiency<br>325–500 mg every 4 h or 500–1000 mg every 6 h<br>Maximum daily dose: per McNeil Consumer Healthcare, 3000 mg/d; Health care professionals may still prescribe 4000 mg/d and are advised to use their own discretion and clinical judgment | • Consider all sources of acetaminophen (prescription and over the counter) and all routes of administration<br>• Monitoring: check liver function, signs and symptoms of liver injury |

contain information on the risk of heart attack and stroke.[63,64] Continued pharmacovigilance research is needed to better describe the comparative efficacy and safety of NSAID use in older adults.

Given the concerns of adverse drug events, NSAIDs are included throughout the updated 2015 American Geriatrics Society Beers Criteria for Potentially Inappropriate Medication Use in Older Adults.[65] The non–cyclooxygenase-selective NSAIDs are included as a medication class to avoid owing to their increased risk of GI bleeding or peptic ulcer disease in high-risk groups, including those aged greater than 75 years or taking oral or parenteral corticosteroids, anticoagulants, or antiplatelet agents. The recommendation is to avoid chronic use, unless other alternatives are not effective and the patient can take a gastroprotective agent (proton pump inhibitor or misoprostol). Indomethacin is specifically called out for its greater risk of adverse CNS effects. Moreover, NSAIDs (including cyclooxygenase-2 inhibitors) are listed as a drug–disease interaction to avoid in older adults with heart failure and chronic kidney disease (creatinine clearance <30 mL/min). Finally, NSAIDs are listed as having clinically important drug–drug interactions with corticosteroids (oral or parenteral) and warfarin owing to an increased risk of peptic ulcer disease and bleeding.

One approach to reducing adverse drug events associated with NSAIDs is to avoid the use of specific agents that are known to interact with NSAIDs and use preferred alternative analgesics (eg, topicals, APAP), sometimes in combination. This is particularly important in older adults with preexisting hypertension, chronic kidney disease, heart failure, and/or peptic ulcer disease, or those taking concomitant warfarin or corticosteroids. If NSAID use is not contraindicated, a trial (eg, 1–2 weeks in duration) of analgesic dosing of a nonacetylated salicylate (eg, salsalate) or ibuprofen or celecoxib may be acceptable.[66] For those with moderate to moderately severe OA pain, a trial of a low-dose opioid or an opioidlike agent (eg, codeine, tramadol) in combination with APAP is another option. The rationale for this approach is to combine 2 different mechanisms of analgesic action. In those older adults who require chronic NSAIDs, a proton pump inhibitor or misoprostol should be used to avoid the risk of peptic ulcer disease.[66] Until further research and guidelines are published on the use of NSAIDs in older adults, clinicians and patients should practice shared decision making to minimize potential risk and maximize patient outcomes from NSAID use (**Table 3**).

## Adjuvant Therapies

Adjuvant pain medications are those that are not typically used as first-line agents for pain, but may be helpful for its management. Agents may be used alone; however, effects are enhanced when used in combination with other analgesics. Currently there are only 2 nonopiate adjuvant therapies approved by the FDA for the treatment of neuropathic pain: pregabalin and duloxetine. Neuropathic pain is characterized by chronic pain, and results from various heterogeneous diagnoses/etiologies (ie, diabetic peripheral neuropathy, postherpetic neuralgia, central post stroke pain, phantom limb pain).[67,68] Therefore, individuals with neuropathic pain and refractory persistent pain whose neuropathic pain is not well-managed with conventional therapies are ideal candidates. As discussed in another section of this series (see Christopher Eccleston and colleagues' article, "Psychological Approaches in Geriatric Pain Management," in this issue), older adults with chronic pain have a substantially increased risk for depression and that depression may intensify a patient's sensitivity to pain.[69,70] Thus, antidepressant use may have synergistic effects in older adults experiencing depression along with chronic pain.[71]

| Table 3 NSAIDs | | | |
|---|---|---|---|
| **Medication** | **Indication** | **Dosage Range** | **Clinical Pearls** |
| Ibuprofen (Motrin) | Mild-to-moderate pain | Consider reduced initial dosage in frailty Renally adjust doses 200 mg 3–4 times per day; maximum daily dose of 3200 mg; administer after meal; if longer term use (eg, >1 mo), GI protection recommended | • Inexpensive<br>• Side effects may be limited by using the lowest effective recommended dose for the shortest time possible |
| Celecoxib (Celebrex) | Mild-to-moderate pain | 100–200 mg/d | • More expensive than other NSAIDs<br>• Higher doses associated with higher incidence of GI and CV side effects; patients with indications for cardioprotection require aspirin<br>• Side effects may be limited by using the lowest effective recommended dose for the shortest time possible |
| Salsalate (Disalcid) | Mild-to-moderate pain | 500–750 mg every 12 h; maximum daily dose of 3000 mg | • Does not interfere with platelet function; GI bleeding and nephrotoxicity are rare<br>• Side effects may be limited by using the lowest effective recommended dose for the shortest time possible |

*Abbreviations:* CV, cardiovascular; GI, gastrointestinal; NSAIDs, nonsteroidal anti-inflammatory drugs.

## Antidepressants

The mechanism for how antidepressants are effective in pain management is not fully known; however, these medications work through the inhibition of neurotransmitter (ie, serotonin and norepinephrine) reuptake in the synaptic cleft,[72] particularly along the descending spinal pain pathways.[68] It is also believed that antidepressants may exert adjunctive therapeutic effects via histamine receptors and sodium channels.[73]

Several antidepressants are efficacious in the management of chronic neuropathic pain, including the tricyclic antidepressants, particularly tertiary amine subtypes, such as amitriptyline, nortriptyline, and doxepin. Despite having the strongest evidence for neuropathy-related pain relief, this class should be avoided in older adults if possible owing to increased risk for adverse effects such as anticholinergic effects and cognitive impairment.[65]

Serotonin–norepinephrine reuptake inhibitors, such as venlafaxine and duloxetine, are mixed acting antidepressants that predominately inhibit serotonin reuptake at low doses and norepinephrine reuptake at high doses, thus increasing these neurotransmitters and dampening pain signals to the brain. Serotonin–norepinephrine reuptake inhibitors are generally well-tolerated by older adults and have fewer side effects compared with tricyclic antidepressants.[74] Venlafaxine has been studied for analgesia with pain relief occurring at higher doses ranging up to 225 mg/d. In a study by Rowbotham and colleagues,[75] 56% of the participants receiving venlafaxine 150 to 225 mg achieved at least a 50% reduction in pain intensity versus 34% of participants in the placebo group. The number needed to treat for an additional beneficial outcome in reduction of pain intensity was 4.5.[75,76] Unfortunately, increased hypertensive episodes have also been noted at these doses. Therefore, the practicality of venlafaxine as an adjunctive agent in neuropathic pain or dual therapy for depression may be limited in older adults.[74] Conversely, duloxetine does not have such effects on blood pressure and is noted to reduce diabetic peripheral neuropathic pain (DPNP) by 50% as compared with placebo.[77]

### Antiepileptics

Anticonvulsants, initially indicated for epileptic seizures with a variety of mechanisms of action, have been shown to be effective at treating various chronic pain conditions, in particular neuropathic pain.[78] Carbamazepine is a prototypical anticonvulsant that blocks voltage-sensitive sodium channels, resulting in the stabilization of hyperexcited neural membranes and inhibition of repetitive firing or reduction of propagation of synaptic impulses.[78] In several studies, carbamazepine has shown efficacy in the treatment of trigeminal neuralgia; however, its use is complicated by pharmacokinetic factors and frequent adverse effects. Within the guidelines for the treatment of neuropathic pain, carbamazepine is listed as a first-line therapy alongside oxcarbazepine, which is noted to have a better side effect profile. However, there are no controlled trials documenting a beneficial effect of oxcarbazepine for trigeminal neuralgia and thus it carries and off-label indication for neuropathic pain.[78,79] If a patient is unable to tolerate carbamazepine, it is reasonable to consider a trial of lamotrigine, which also has shown efficacy in trigeminal neuralgia by stabilizing sodium channels and suppressing the release of glutamate.[78]

Gabapentin and pregabalin are modulators of the alpha-2-delta subunit of the calcium channels in the CNS, accounting for antinociceptive and antiepileptic effects. Gabapentin is indicated for PHN; although not FDA indicated in the treatment of DPNP, it has demonstrated efficacy for this condition and is widely used in clinical practice.[79–81] Gabapentin shows similar efficacy in pain reduction to pregabalin, with a number needed to treat of 3.9 to 4.2; however, pregabalin is FDA indicated for PHN, DPNP, and fibromyalgia.[82,83] In a study conducted in older adults (mean age 66 years), both anticonvulsants have consistently shown improvement in mood, sleep disturbance, and quality of life.[81] When compared with antidepressants such as duloxetine and amitriptyline on the primary outcome of subjective pain, there is no difference among treatment groups (amitriptyline, duloxetine, pregabalin) in the reduction of pain severity.[81] In a study[84] comparing duloxetine versus pregabalin versus duloxetine and gabapentin in patients (mean age, 61 years) with DPNP, there were no between-group differences with respect to treatment emergent events (including nausea, vomiting, insomnia, peripheral edema, hyperhidrosis, or decreased appetite). Insomnia was reported more frequently in the pregabalin and gabapentin groups.[84] In the older adult population, there was an increased risk for falls with the use of gabapentin and pregabalin owing mainly to the side effects of dizziness and somnolence. Of note, the 2015 AGS Beers Criteria[65] identify both agents as potentially inappropriate medications in older adults with a history of falls or fractures (unless being used for the treatment of seizure or mood disorders). The updated criteria recommend increased monitoring with renal impairment. Because both agents are primarily excreted renally, dose adjustment should be considered as renal function declines[65] (**Table 4**).

**Table 4**
**Adjuvant therapies**

| Medication | Indication | Dosage Range | Clinical Pearls |
|---|---|---|---|
| **Antidepressants** | | | |
| Amitriptyline (Elavil) | Diabetic peripheral neuropathy (off-label) | Start 10 mg/d Titrate at tolerated, lower doses are recommended | Caution anticholinergic effects/burden |
| Nortriptyline (Pamelor) | Diabetic peripheral neuropathy (off-label) Postherpetic neuralgia (off-label) | Start 10–20 mg/d (bedtime) Titrate every 3–5 d as tolerated in 10 mg increments Max 160 mg/d | • Fewer anticholinergic effects than other tricyclic antidepressants<br>• Preferred in older adult population; however, still need to monitor for anticholinergic effects/burden |
| Venlafaxine ER (Effexor XR) | Diabetic peripheral neuropathy (off-label) | Start 37.5 mg/d Titrate to 75–225 mg/d | • Monitor blood pressure, and for increased anxiety or insomnia<br>• May impair platelet aggregation, monitor for bruising and bleeding<br>• Associated with hyponatremia, monitor sodium levels upon initiation, dose changes and periodically during therapy |
| Duloxetine (Cymbalta) | Diabetic peripheral neuropathy Fibromyalgia | Start 30–60 mg/d Titrate to 60–120 mg/d | • Preferred SNRI for older adults<br>• Well tolerated with reduced incidence of SNRI typical side effects<br>• Association with hyponatremia remains the same as other SNRIs |
| **Anticonvulsants** | | | |
| Carbamazepine (Tegretol) | Trigeminal neuralgia | Start 200 mg/d BID Titrate to 400–800 mg/d BID | • Several drug interactions<br>• Nausea, edema, insomnia, agitation, Stevens–Johnson syndrome |
| Oxcarbazepine (Trileptal) | Trigeminal neuralgia (off-label use) | Start 300–600 mg/d BID Titrate to 1500–1800 mg/d BID | Elevated blood pressure, dizziness, drowsiness, headache, agitation, nausea, constipation, vomiting |
| Lamotrigine (Lamictal) | Trigeminal neuralgia | Start 5 mg/d Titrate to 200–600 mg/d | Monitor for hypersensitivity reactions, (rash, acute urticarial, and extensive pruritus); risk is higher with the coadministration of valproic acid |

*(continued on next page)*

**Table 4**
*(continued)*

| Medication | Indication | Dosage Range | Clinical Pearls |
|---|---|---|---|
| Gabapentin (Neurontin) | Postherpetic neuralgia<br>Diabetic peripheral neuropathy (off-label)<br>Fibromyalgia (off-label) | Start 300 mg/d TID<br>Titrate to 1800–3600 mg/d TID | • Monitor renal function as gabapentin should be dose adjusted when CrCl <60 mL/min<br>• Caution increased risk for falls due to dizziness and somnolence |
| Pregabalin (Lyrica) | Postherpetic neuralgia<br>Diabetic peripheral neuropathy<br>Fibromyalgia | Start 150 mg/d BID-TID<br>Titrate to 150–300 mg/d BID–TID | • Controlled substance C-IV<br>• Monitor renal function as gabapentin should be dose adjusted when CrCl <60 mL/min<br>• Caution increased risk for falls due to dizziness and somnolence |

*Abbreviations:* BID, twice a day; CrCl, creatinine clearance; SNRI, serotonin-norepinephrine reuptake inhibitors; TID, 3 times a day.

### Muscle Relaxants

Skeletal muscle relaxants include a variety of agents that are separated into 2 categories: antispasticity agents and antispasmodics.[85] Each of these categories has different indications, mechanisms of action, and side effect profiles. Antispasticity agents work on the spinal cord or directly on the skeletal muscle to improve hypertonicity and involuntary spasms. These medications are used for spastic conditions such as cerebral palsy, multiple sclerosis, spinal cord injuries and after cerebrovascular accidents; this category of medications should be used with caution in older adults with chronic pain due to degenerative or neuropathic pain. The use of skeletal muscle relaxants among older adults is associated with sedation and confusion, which may lead to an increased risk of falls and injuries.[86] Per the 2015 Beers criteria, muscle relaxants (including cyclobenzaprine, carisoprodol, methocarbamol, and metaxolone) are considered as being high-risk medications in older adults due to anticholinergic adverse drug effects, excessive sedation, and weakness; however, they continue to be used among older adults.[65] Further, a recent retrospective cohort study in older (>65 years of age) Veterans showed that muscle relaxants (including methocarbamol and cyclobenzaprine, among others) were associated with increased risk for emergency department visits as well as all-cause hospitalizations (including those for falls and fractures).[87] Another commonly used agent used for spasticity, and not included in the Beer's criteria, is baclofen. Baclofen is a centrally acting skeletal muscle relaxant with an FDA indication to treat spasticity related to CNS lesions; dosing regimens vary by indication. Among the antispasticity agents, baclofen is generally well-tolerated with a decreased occurrence of CNS depression. Dantrolene is another agent that works peripherally to increase the release of calcium from the sarcoplasmic reticulum in the skeletal muscle cell thus slowing contraction cycles. However, use of dantrolene is limited by the risk of hepatotoxicity with chronic use. Last, tizanidine is a centrally acting alpha 2-adrenergic agonist that increases the inhibition of presynaptic motor neurons with no direct effect on muscle fibers. Similarly, its use in older adults is limited by dose-dependent adverse drug events, drug–drug interactions, and the possibility of prolonged QT intervals (**Table 5**).

**Table 5**
**Muscle relaxants**

| Medication | Indication | Dosage Range | Clinical Pearls |
|---|---|---|---|
| **Antispasticity Agents** | | | |
| Baclofen (Lioresal) | Spasticity | 5 mg 2–3 times/d for Max 80 mg/d | • Black box warning: Caution abrupt discontinuation, risk of withdrawal<br>• No dose adjustments required for renal or hepatic dysfunction |
| Dantrolene (Dantrium) | Spasticity | Start 25 mg (25–100 mg) 4 times/d | • Black bock warning: risk for hepatotoxicity with chronic use, monitor hepatic function<br>• May cause sun sensitivity |
| Tizanidine (Zanaflex) | Spasticity | Initial 2 mg ≤3 times/d Titrate in 2-4 mg increments per dose over 1–4 d Max 36 mg/d (single doses of >16 mg have not been studied) | • Avoid rapid discontinuation: gradually taper by 2-4 mg/d<br>• Use with caution in older adults who have decreased clearance<br>• Monitor liver function<br>• Monitor QT interval with chronic use |
| **Antispasmodic agents** | | | |
| Carisoprodol (Soma) | Acute musculoskeletal pain | 250–350 mg 3 times/d | • Controlled substance C-IV has been subject to abuse, dependence, withdrawal, misuse, and diversion<br>• Active metabolites with barbiturate effects increasing somnolence and risk of falls for older adults<br>• Caution orthostatic hypotension<br>• Limit use to 2–3 wk |
| Cyclobenzaprine (Amrix; Flexeril DSC) | Musculoskeletal pain | IR tablet 5 mg 3 times/d Max 10 mg 3 times/d Extended-release tables – not recommended for geriatric patients | • Caution anticholinergic effects/burden<br>• Not recommended in mild to severe hepatic impairment<br>• Do not use within 14 d of MAOIs |
| Metaxolone (Skelaxin) | Musculoskeletal pain | 800 mg 3–4 times/d | • Absorption is increased when taken with food<br>• Contraindicated in severe hepatic and renal dysfunction, monitor liver function |

*(continued on next page)*

| Table 5 (*continued*) | | | |
|---|---|---|---|
| **Medication** | **Indication** | **Dosage Range** | **Clinical Pearls** |
| Methocarbamol (Robaxin) | Musculoskeletal pain | 750–1000 mg orally every 4 hours, up to 4 g/day for maintenance<br>Max 4 g/d | • Use lower doses at initiation of drug especially with geriatric patients, titrate as clinically indicated<br>• No dose adjustments required for renal or hepatic dysfunction<br>• Drug may change color of urine to brown, black, or green |

*Abbreviations:* IR, immediate release; MAOI, monoamine oxidase inhibitors.

### New Analgesics in the Pipeline

The medication classes discussed in this article are traditionally known to be first-, second-, or third-line agents for chronic pain. There are many new agents and compounds in varying stages of development/testing for the treatment of chronic pain (eg, angiotensin II receptor antagonist, calcitonin gene-related peptide). At this time, it is premature to predict the potential role of these newer medications for chronic pain management in older adults. In the absence of new safe and effective analgesics, the primary focus is to trial existing therapies, in different combinations, and with different multidisciplinary approaches to maximize pain relief and minimize medication toxicity.

### Making a Plan: Approach to Managing Chronic Pain in Older Adults with Pharmacologic Agents

#### Expectations and treatment goals

"Success" is determined largely by whether treatment goals, established jointly by the patient and provider, are met.[71] The older adult should be encouraged to communicate his/her expectations for pain relief. The field of pain management is moving away from solely assessing and managing a pain intensity score (eg, a 0–10 numeric rating score) and toward understanding and targeting the functional outcomes and personal (realistic) goals that older adults would like to achieve.

#### Monitoring and managing medication adjustments for older adults

The clinical challenge is how to manage pain effectively and safely in older adults. Many older adults have already tried several classes of medications and may be hesitant to attempt a trial of a new medication or a combination of analgesics. Using 2 or more analgesic medications with complementary mechanisms of action may lead to greater pain relief with less toxicity as opposed to higher doses of a single pain medication. Starting 1 medication at a time is a preferred strategy to better evaluate effect and safety. Several strategies may help providers to achieve success when recommending new analgesic trials or combinations of therapy:

- Be prepared to respond to questions and concerns for each medication or combination thereof;

- Provide potential options for "rescue" pain medications during trials of new medications;
- Be available to listen to and be receptive to the patients' concerns;
- Avoid communicating guarantees of positive results;
- Emphasize the need for adherence to the instructed regimen;
- Encourage the patient to call if new concerning signs or symptoms develop after starting the medication;
- Develop a careful surveillance plan to determine whether treatment goals are being met and for monitoring potential toxicity; and
- If goals are not met, consider tapering and discontinuing medication.[10,29]

To achieve patient identified therapeutic goals (including reduction in pain intensity and pain related disability) with pharmacologic (and/or nonpharmacological) management, employing a multidisciplinary approach is paramount. Thus, successful pain management in older adults requires a collaborative approach among all members of the health care team. Finally, combining pharmacologic and nonpharmacological (including activity based, psychological) interventions is likely to have the highest yield for improving pain control in older adults.

## REFERENCES

1. Blyth FM, March LM, Brnabic AJ, et al. Chronic pain in Australia: a prevalence study. Pain 2001;89:127–34.
2. Elliott AM, Smith BH, Penny KI, et al. The epidemiology of chronic pain in the community. Lancet 1999;354:1248–52.
3. Gaskin DJ, Richard P. The economic costs of pain in the United States. J Pain 2012;13:715–24.
4. Helme RD, Gibson SJ. The epidemiology of pain in elderly people. Clin Geriatr Med 2001;17:417–31.
5. Katz JN. Lumbar disc disorders and low-back pain: socioeconomic factors and consequences. J Bone Joint Surg Am 2006;88(Suppl 2):21–4.
6. Patel KV, Guralnik JM, Dansie EJ, et al. Prevalence and impact of pain among older adults in the United States: findings from the 2011 National Health and Aging Trends Study. Pain 2013;154:2649–57.
7. Lawrence RC, Helmick CG, Arnett FC, et al. Estimates of the prevalence of arthritis and selected musculoskeletal disorders in the United States. Arthritis Rheum 1998;41:778–99.
8. Buchman AS, Shah RC, Leurgans SE, et al. Musculoskeletal pain and incident disability in community-dwelling older adults. Arthritis Care Res 2010;62:1287–93.
9. Whitson HE, Landerman LR, Newman AB, et al. Chronic medical conditions and the sex-based disparity in disability: the Cardiovascular Health Study. J Gerontol A Biol Sci Med Sci 2010;65:1325–31.
10. Abdulla A, Adams N, Bone M, et al. Guidance on the management of pain in older people. Age Ageing 2013;42(Suppl 1):i1–57.
11. Reid MC, Williams CS, Gill TM. The relationship between psychological factors and disabling musculoskeletal pain in community-dwelling older persons. J Am Geriatr Soc 2003;51:1092–8.
12. Leveille SG, Ling S, Hochberg MC, et al. Widespread musculoskeletal pain and the progression of disability in older disabled women. Ann Intern Med 2001;135:1038–46.

13. Leveille SG, Bean J, Ngo L, et al. The pathway from musculoskeletal pain to mobility difficulty in older disabled women. Pain 2007;128:69–77.
14. Buchner M, Neubauer E, Zahlten-Hinguranage A, et al. Age as a predicting factor in the therapy outcome of multidisciplinary treatment of patients with chronic low back pain - a prospective longitudinal clinical study in 405 patients. Clin Rheumatol 2007;26:385–92.
15. Reid MC, Bennett DA, Chen WG, et al. Improving the pharmacologic management of pain in older adults: identifying the research gaps and methods to address them. Pain Med 2011;12:1336–57.
16. Institute of Medicine. Relieving pain in America: a blueprint for transforming prevention, care, education, and research. Washington, DC: National Academic Press; 2011.
17. Spitz A, Moore AA, Papaleontiou M, et al. Primary care providers' perspective on prescribing opioids to older adults with chronic non-cancer pain: a qualitative study. BMC Geriatr 2011;11:35.
18. Thielke S, Sale J, Reid MC. Aging: are these 4 pain myths complicating care? J Fam Pract 2012;61:666–70.
19. Paeck T, Ferreira ML, Sun C, et al. Are older adults missing from low back pain clinical trials? A systematic review and meta-analysis. Arthritis Care Res 2014; 66:1220–6.
20. Jadad AR, To MJ, Emara M, et al. Consideration of multiple chronic diseases in randomized controlled trials. JAMA 2011;306:2670–2.
21. Marcum ZA, Gurwitz JH, Colon-Emeric C, et al. Pills and ills: methodological problems in pharmacological research. J Am Geriatr Soc 2015;63: 829–30.
22. Tinetti ME, Fried TR, Boyd CM. Designing health care for the most common chronic condition–multimorbidity. JAMA 2012;307:2493–4.
23. Shavers VL, Bakos A, Sheppard VB. Race, ethnicity, and pain among the U.S. adult population. J Health Care Poor Underserved 2010;21:177–220.
24. Anderson KO, Green CR, Payne R. Racial and ethnic disparities in pain: causes and consequences of unequal care. J Pain 2009;10:1187–204.
25. Green CR, Anderson KO, Baker TA, et al. The unequal burden of pain: confronting racial and ethnic disparities in pain. Pain Med 2003;4:277–94.
26. Hadjistavropoulos T, Herr K, Turk DC, et al. An interdisciplinary expert consensus statement on assessment of pain in older persons. Clin J Pain 2007;23:S1–43.
27. Pergolizzi J, Böger RH, Budd K, et al. Opioids and the management of chronic severe pain in the elderly: consensus statement of an international expert panel with focus on the six clinically most often used World Health Organization step III Opioids (Buprenorphine, Fentanyl, Hydromorphone, Methadone, Morphine, Oxycodone). Pain Pract 2008;8:287–313.
28. AGS Panel on Persistent Pain in Older Persons. The management of persistent pain in older persons. J Am Geriatr Soc 2002;50(6 Suppl): S205–24.
29. American Geriatrics Society Panel on Pharmacological Management of Persistent Pain in Older Persons. Pharmacological management of persistent pain in older persons. J Am Geriatr Soc 2009;57(8):1331–46.
30. Fried TR, Tinetti ME, Iannone L, et al. Health outcome prioritization as a tool for decision making among older persons with multiple chronic conditions. Arch Intern Med 2011;171:1854–6.

31. Dobscha SK, Corson K, Perrin NA, et al. Collaborative care for chronic pain in primary care: a cluster randomized trial. JAMA 2009;301:1242–52.
32. Dowell D, Haegerich TM, Chou R. CDC guideline for prescribing opioids for chronic pain - United States, 2016. MMWR Recomm Rep 2016;65(RR-1):1–49.
33. Dowell D, Haegerich TM, Chou R. CDC Guideline for prescribing opioids for chronic pain - United States, 2016. JAMA 2016;315(15):1624–56.
34. Argoff CE, Viscusi ER. The use of opioid analgesics for chronic pain: minimizing the risk for harm. Am J Gastroenterol 2014;2:3–8.
35. Kaestli LZ, Wasilewski-Rasca AF, Bonnabry P, et al. Use of transdermal drug formulations in the elderly. Drugs Aging 2008;25:269–80.
36. Topp R, Brosky JA Jr, Pieschel D. The effect of either topical menthol or a placebo on functioning and knee pain among patients with knee OA. J Geriatr Phys Ther 2013;36:92–9.
37. Mou J, Paillard F, Turnbull B, et al. Efficacy of Qutenza(R) (capsaicin) 8% patch for neuropathic pain: a meta-analysis of the Qutenza Clinical Trials Database. Pain 2013;154:1632–9.
38. Pasero C. Lidocaine patch 5% for acute pain management. J Perianesth Nurs 2013;28:169–73.
39. Rains C, Bryson HM. Topical capsaicin. A review of its pharmacological properties and therapeutic potential in post-herpetic neuralgia, diabetic neuropathy and osteoarthritis. Drugs Aging 1995;7:317–28.
40. Derry S, Sven-Rice A, Cole P, et al. Topical capsaicin (high concentration) for chronic neuropathic pain in adults. Cochrane Database Syst Rev 2013;(2):CD007393.
41. Treatment of painful diabetic neuropathy with topical capsaicin. A multicenter, double-blind, vehicle-controlled study. The Capsaicin Study Group. Arch Intern Med 1991;151:2225–9.
42. Deal CL, Schnitzer TJ, Lipstein E, et al. Treatment of arthritis with topical capsaicin: a double-blind trial. Clin Ther 1991;13:383–95.
43. Peikert A, Hentrich M, Ochs G. Topical 0.025% capsaicin in chronic post-herpetic neuralgia: efficacy, predictors of response and long-term course. J Neurol 1991;238:452–6.
44. Zacher J, Altman R, Bellamy N, et al. Topical diclofenac and its role in pain and inflammation: an evidence-based review. Curr Med Res Opin 2008;24:925–50.
45. Mason L, Moore R, Edwards J, et al. Topical NSAIDs for chronic musculoskeletal pain: systematic review and meta-analysis. BMC Musculoskelet Disord 2004;5:28.
46. Tugwell P, Wells G, Shainhouse J. Equivalence study of a topical diclofenac solution (Pennsaid) compared with oral diclofenac in symptomatic treatment of osteoarthritis of the knee: a randomized controlled trial. J Rheumatol 2004;31:2002–12.
47. Underwood M, Ashby D, Cross P, et al. Advice to use topical or oral ibuprofen for chronic knee pain in older people: randomised controlled trial and patient preference study. BMJ 2008;336:138–42.
48. Fraenkel L, Wittink DR, Concato J, et al. Informed choice and the widespread use of antiinflammatory drugs. Arthritis Rheum 2004;51:210–4.
49. Makris UE, Kohler MJ, Fraenkel L. Adverse effects of topical nonsteroidal antiinflammatory drugs in older adults with osteoarthritis: a systematic literature review. J Rheumatol 2010;37:1236–43.

50. O'Neil CK, Hanlon JT, Marcum ZA. Adverse effects of analgesics commonly used by older adults with osteoarthritis: focus on non-opioid and opioid analgesics. Am J Geriatr Pharmacother 2012;10:331–42.

51. Moyer RF, Hunter DJ. Osteoarthritis in 2014: changing how we define and treat patients with OA. Nat Rev Rheumatol 2015;11:65–6.

52. Bannuru RR, Schmid CH, Kent DM, et al. Comparative effectiveness of pharmacologic interventions for knee osteoarthritis: a systematic review and network meta-analysis. Ann Intern Med 2015;162:46–54.

53. Machado GC, Maher CG, Ferreira PH, et al. Efficacy and safety of paracetamol for spinal pain and osteoarthritis: systematic review and meta-analysis of randomised placebo controlled trials. BMJ 2015;350:h1225.

54. Roberts E, Delgado Nunes V, Buckner S, et al. Paracetamol: not as safe as we thought? A systematic literature review of observational studies. Ann Rheum Dis 2015;75(3):552–9.

55. Kennelty KA, Parmelee P, Wilson NL. From policy to practice: an interdisciplinary look at recent FDA policy changes for acetaminophen and the implications for patient care. Washington, DC: The Gerontological Society of America; 2015.

56. Deveza LA, Hunter DJ. Pain relief for an osteoarthritic knee in the elderly: a practical guide. Drugs Aging 2016;33:11–20.

57. Hanlon JT, Fillenbaum GG, Studenski SA, et al. Factors associated with suboptimal analgesic use in community-dwelling elderly. Ann Pharmacother 1996;30:739–44.

58. Griffin MR. Epidemiology of nonsteroidal anti-inflammatory drug-associated gastrointestinal injury. Am J Med 1998;104:23S–9S [discussion: 41S–2S].

59. Gupta M, Eisen GM. NSAIDs and the gastrointestinal tract. Curr Gastroenterol Rep 2009;11:345–53.

60. Ray WA, Stein CM, Byrd V, et al. Educational program for physicians to reduce use of non-steroidal anti-inflammatory drugs among community-dwelling elderly persons: a randomized controlled trial. Med Care 2001;39:425–35.

61. Hanlon JT, Guay DRP, Ives TJ. Oral analgesics: efficacy, mechanism of action, pharmacokinetics, adverse effects, and practical recommendations for use in older adults. In: Gibson SJ, Weiner DK, editors. Pain in older persons. Seattle (WA): IASP Press; 2005. p. 205–22.

62. McGettigan P, Henry D. Cardiovascular risk with non-steroidal anti-inflammatory drugs: systematic review of population-based controlled observational studies. PLoS Med 2011;8:e1001098.

63. FDA strengthens warning that non-aspirin nonsteroidal anti-inflammatory drugs (NSAIDs) can cause heart attacks or strokes [Internet]. 2015. Available at: http://www.fda.gov/Drugs/DrugSafety/ucm451800.htm. Accessed July 25, 2015.

64. FDA Briefing Information for the February 10-11, 2014 Joint Meeting of the Arthritis Advisory Committee and Drug Safety and Risk Management Advisory Committee. [Internet]. Available at: http://www.fda.gov/downloads/Advisory Committees/CommitteesMeetingMaterials/Drugs/ArthritisAdvisoryCommittee/UCM 383180.pdf.2014. Accessed July 25, 2016.

65. By the American Geriatrics Society Beers Criteria Update Expert Panel. American Geriatrics Society 2015 updated beers criteria for potentially inappropriate medication use in older adults. J Am Geriatr Soc 2015;63:2227–46.

66. Marcum ZA, Hanlon JT. Recognizing the risks of chronic nonsteroidal anti-inflammatory drug use in older adults. Ann Longterm Care 2010;18: 24–7.
67. Kaye AD, Baluch A, Scott JT. Pain management in the elderly population: a review. Ochsner J 2010;10:179–87.
68. Sansone RA, Sansone LA. Pain, pain, go away: antidepressants and pain management. Psychiatry (Edgmont) 2008;5:16–9.
69. Gagliese L, Melzack R. Chronic pain in elderly people. Pain 1997;70:3–14.
70. Hanssen DJ, Naarding P, Collard RM, et al. Physical, lifestyle, psychological, and social determinants of pain intensity, pain disability, and the number of pain locations in depressed older adults. Pain 2014;155:2088–96.
71. Makris UE, Abrams RC, Gurland B, et al. Management of persistent pain in the older patient: a clinical review. JAMA 2014;312:825–36.
72. Kapur BM, Lala PK, Shaw JL. Pharmacogenetics of chronic pain management. Clin Biochem 2014;47:1169–87.
73. Gallagher RM. Management of neuropathic pain: translating mechanistic advances and evidence-based research into clinical practice. Clin J Pain 2006; 22:S2–8.
74. Duncan NA, Mahan RJ, Turner SJ. Non-opiate pharmacotherapy options for the management of pain in older adults. Mental Health Clinician 2015;5(3):91–101.
75. Rowbotham MC, Goli V, Kunz NR, et al. Venlafaxine extended release in the treatment of painful diabetic neuropathy: a double-blind, placebo-controlled study. Pain 2004;110:697–706.
76. Gallagher HC, Gallagher RM, Butler M, et al. Venlafaxine for neuropathic pain in adults. Cochrane Database Syst Rev 2015;(8):CD011091.
77. Peltier A, Goutman SA, Callaghan BC. Painful diabetic neuropathy. BMJ 2014; 348:g1799.
78. Jensen TS. Anticonvulsants in neuropathic pain: rationale and clinical evidence. Eur J Pain 2002;6(Suppl A):61–8.
79. Bril V, England J, Franklin GM, et al. Evidence-based guideline: treatment of painful diabetic neuropathy: report of the American Academy of Neurology, the American Association of Neuromuscular and Electrodiagnostic Medicine, and the American Academy of Physical Medicine and Rehabilitation. Neurology 2011; 76:1758–65.
80. Dworkin RH, O'Connor AB, Backonja M, et al. Pharmacologic management of neuropathic pain: evidence-based recommendations. Pain 2007;132: 237–51.
81. Boyle J, Eriksson MEV, Gribble L, et al. Randomized, placebo-controlled comparison of amitriptyline, duloxetine, and pregabalin in patients with chronic diabetic peripheral neuropathic pain: impact on pain, polysomnographic sleep, daytime functioning, and quality of life. Diabetes Care 2012;35:2451–8.
82. Quilici S, Chancellor J, Lothgren M, et al. Meta-analysis of duloxetine vs. pregabalin and gabapentin in the treatment of diabetic peripheral neuropathic pain. BMC Neurol 2009;9:6.
83. Ziegler D, Fonseca V. From guideline to patient: a review of recent recommendations for pharmacotherapy of painful diabetic neuropathy. J Diabet Complications 2015;29:146–56.
84. Irving G, Tanenberg RJ, Raskin J, et al. Comparative safety and tolerability of duloxetine vs. pregabalin vs. duloxetine plus gabapentin in patients with diabetic peripheral neuropathic pain. Int J Clin Pract 2014;68:1130–40.

85. Witenko C, Moorman-Li R, Motycka C, et al. Considerations for the appropriate use of skeletal muscle relaxants for the management of acute low back pain. P T 2014;39:427–35.

86. Spence MM, Shin PJ, Lee EA, et al. Risk of injury associated with skeletal muscle relaxant use in older adults. Ann Pharmacother 2013;47:993–8.

87. Makris UE, Pugh MJ, Alvarez CA, et al. Exposure to high-risk medications is associated with worse outcomes in older Veterans with chronic pain. Am J Med Sci 2015;350:279–85.

## APPENDIX 1: RECOMMENDED RESOURCES FOR PHARMACOLOGIC MANAGEMENT OF CHRONIC PAIN IN OLDER ADULTS

| Resource | Content | Origin | Last Updated |
|---|---|---|---|
| American College of Rheumatology (ACR) | Practice guidelines for the treatment of osteoarthritis (hand, hip, and knee) | USA | 2012 |
| American Geriatrics Society (AGS) | Practice guideline for pharmacologic management of chronic pain | USA | 2009 |
| National Institute for Health and Care Excellence (NICE) | Guidance on the management of chronic pain | UK | 2013 |
| American Geriatrics Society Beers Criteria for Potentially Inappropriate Prescribing in Older Adults | Evidence-based consensus guidelines on potentially inappropriate medication use in older adults, including analgesics | USA | 2015 |
| Osteoarthritis Research Society International (OARSI) Guidelines | Guidelines for the management of hip and knee osteoarthritis | Global | 2014 (knee); 2010 (hip and knee) |
| Center for Disease Control and Prevention (CDC) | Guidelines for prescribing opioids for chronic pain | USA | 2016 |

# The Role of Opioid Analgesics in Geriatric Pain Management

Jennifer Greene Naples, PharmD[a], Walid F. Gellad, MD, MPH[b,c],
Joseph T. Hanlon, PharmD, MS[d,*]

## KEYWORDS

- Opioid • Aged • Pharmacokinetics • Adverse drug event

## KEY POINTS

- Opioids remain a treatment option for moderate to severe chronic noncancer pain when nonopioid analgesics and nonpharmacologic therapies do not provide adequate relief.
- Age-related changes in pharmacokinetics (decreases in hepatic and renal function) and pharmacodynamics make older adults more susceptible to adverse consequences associated with opioids, including falls, fractures, and delirium.
- To optimize the use of opioids, avoid those that have not been studied in older adults.
- Start with the lowest available dose of an immediate-release product, and consult pharmacists or pain experts for challenging cases, including those requiring high doses.

## INTRODUCTION

When possible, chronic noncancer pain (CNCP) in older adults should be managed by nonpharmacologic modalities in conjunction with nonopioid analgesics. If moderate-to-severe pain persists despite these approaches, however, nonparenteral opioids

Disclosures: Dr J.G. Naples's fellowship is supported by a National Institute on Aging grant (T32-AG021885). Dr J.T. Hanlon is supported by National Institute of Aging grants (P30AG024827 and R01AG037451), a grant from the Donoghue Foundation, a grant from the Agency for Healthcare Research and Quality (R18 HS023779), and VA Health Services Research and Development (HSR&D) Service Merit awards (IIR 12-379 and 1 I01 HX001765). Dr W.F. Gellad is supported by VA HSR&D award I01 HX001765.
[a] Division of Geriatrics & Gerontology, Department of Medicine, University of Pittsburgh School of Medicine, University of Pittsburgh, 3471 Fifth Avenue, Kaufmann Medical Building Suite 500, Pittsburgh, PA 15213, USA; [b] Center for Health Equity Research and Promotion, VA Pittsburgh Healthcare System, University of Pittsburgh, Pittsburgh, PA, USA; [c] Division of General Medicine, Department of Medicine, University of Pittsburgh School of Medicine, University Drive (151C), Pittsburgh, PA 15240, USA; [d] Center for Health Equity Research and Promotion, Geriatric Research Education and Clinical Center, VA Pittsburgh Healthcare System, University of Pittsburgh, 3471 Fifth Avenue, Kaufmann Medical Building Suite 500, Pittsburgh, PA 15213, USA
* Corresponding author.
E-mail address: jth14@pitt.edu

Clin Geriatr Med 32 (2016) 725–735
http://dx.doi.org/10.1016/j.cger.2016.06.006
0749-0690/16/© 2016 Elsevier Inc. All rights reserved.

(**Box 1**) may be considered as adjunctive therapy.[1,2] This article reviews the epidemiology of opioid use and their effectiveness for CNCP in older adults, and summarizes important age-related changes in opioid pharmacokinetics and pharmacodynamics that increase the risks of adverse effects in the elderly. Finally, to assist clinicians with selecting appropriate therapy, the article concludes with an evidence-based approach to optimize opioid prescribing in older adults with CNCP.

## EPIDEMIOLOGY OF OPIOID USE AND TREATMENT BENEFITS FOR CHRONIC NONCANCER PAIN IN OLDER PERSONS

Approximately 6% to 9% of community-dwelling older adults use opioids chronically for CNCP.[6–8] A recent study using data from the National Ambulatory Medical Care Survey showed that from 1999 to 2000 to 2009 to 2010, the percentage of clinic visits for older patients where an opioid was prescribed rose from 4.1% to 9.0%.[9] Most commonly, hydrocodone was used in combination with acetaminophen or ibuprofen.[9] Additionally, women and individuals diagnosed with arthritis and depression were more likely to use opioids.[9] Compared with the community setting, opioid use may be even higher in nursing homes. For example, 1 study found that 70% of nursing home residents with CNCP received regularly scheduled opioids.[10] Interestingly, there may be a difference between practice settings regarding the potency of opioids most often prescribed. One study found that higher potency opioids (eg, oxycodone) were

---

**Box 1**
**Nonparenteral, single-ingredient opioids available in the United States**

*Full μ agonist opioids*

Codeine[d]

Fentanyl[b]

Hydrocodone[c]

Hydromorphone[c]

Levorphanol[b]

Meperidine[d]

Methadone[b]

Morphine[c]

Oxycodone[c]

Oxymorphone[c]

*Partial μ agonist opioid*

Buprenorphine[c]

*Mixed action opioids[a]*

Tapentadol[d]

Tramadol[d]

[a] Mixed action = μ receptor agonist and norepinephrine reuptake inhibitor.
[b] High potency.
[c] Moderate potency.
[d] Low potency.
*Data from* Refs.[3–5]

more likely to be used among nursing home residents, whereas lower potency opioids (eg, tramadol) were more frequently given to community-dwelling older adults.[11]

Unfortunately, data regarding the efficacy of opioids for CNCP in older adults are limited to short-term studies. In a 2010 metaanalysis of 18 randomized, placebo-controlled trials, the majority of studies (78%) focused on opioids for osteoarthritis; the remaining studies evaluated their efficacy for neuropathic pain.[12] The most commonly studied opioids, in rank order, were tramadol (n = 7), oxycodone (n = 5), oxymorphone (n = 3), morphine (n = 2), codeine (n = 1), fentanyl (n = 1), and methadone (n = 1).[12] Overall, pooled data showed a significant small-to-modest improvement in pain intensity and physical function with opioids compared with placebo.[12] Despite documented improvements in CNCP from these short-term studies; however, a recently published systematic review found no rigorously conducted long-term trials comparing opioids with nonopioid analgesics for CNCP with a duration of greater than 1 year.[13] This represents an important gap in current clinical knowledge, because there is concern that many patients who use opioids chronically may still have high pain intensity and poor function.[14]

## AGE-RELATED PHARMACOKINETIC AND PHARMACODYNAMIC CHANGES AND RISKS OF OPIOIDS IN OLDER PERSONS

To ensure benefits and minimize risks associated with opioid use in older adults, it is critical to understand age-related changes in pharmacokinetics that affect opioid absorption, distribution, metabolism, and elimination. Oral absorption, indicated by bioavailability (ie, the proportion of drug that reaches systemic circulation), is similar for younger and older adults. For example, the absorption of transdermal buprenorphine and fentanyl does not seem to be altered, despite age-related changes in the skin.[15,16] An exception is morphine, a drug with high first-pass properties, where older patients have greater oral absorption than their younger counterparts.[17] Moreover, opioid distribution is generally not altered in the elderly, despite age-related changes in body composition.[18,19]

Unlike absorption and distribution, however, age-related changes in metabolism are more apparent. All opioids are metabolized by the liver; **Table 1** lists those opioids that undergo phase I and phase II metabolism via respective isoenzymes. In general, drugs metabolized in phase I via the cytochrome P450 enzyme system will undergo oxidation, reduction, or hydrolysis. Age-related reduction in CYP3A4 function may affect opioids, resulting in decreased systemic clearance and subsequent increased elimination half-life. Specifically, the systemic clearance of oxycodone and, possibly, buprenorphine have been shown to decrease with age.[16,20,21] The effect of age on fentanyl clearance in older adults, however, is unclear.[22] Neither the pharmacokinetics nor efficacy of either methadone or levorphanol have been studied in older adults. Moreover, there are reports of QT interval prolongation with methadone. Therefore, the prescribing by those without extensive clinical experience with these agents is not recommended.[23]

The effect of age on CYP2D6 metabolism is unclear, although it is well-documented that genetic polymorphisms may result in poor, intermediate, extensive, and ultrarapid metabolism.[19,24,25] Theoretically, CYP2D6 poor metabolizers may have reduced efficacy with codeine, hydrocodone, and tramadol, because these medications are prodrugs that require conversion to an active form before exerting their pharmacologic effect (see **Table 1**). However, there is no clinical evidence for any opioids that undergo CYP2D6 metabolism to suggest that dose adjustments for opioids used chronically are required.[25]

**Table 1**
**Hepatic metabolism pathways for opioids**

| Phase | Isoenzyme | Substrate | Active Metabolite |
|-------|-----------|-----------|-------------------|
| I | CYP2D6 | Codeine[a] (prodrug) | Morphine |
|   |   | Hydrocodone[a] (prodrug) | Hydromorphone |
|   |   | Tramadol (prodrug) | O-desmethyltramadol |
|   | CYP3A4 | Buprenorphine | None |
|   |   | Fentanyl | None |
|   |   | Meperidine | Normeperidine |
|   |   | Methadone[a] | None |
|   |   | Oxycodone | Oxymorphone and noroxycodone |
| II | UGT | Hydromorphone | Hydromorphone-3-glucuronide |
|   |   | Levorphanol[a] | None |
|   |   | Morphine | Morphine-3-and 6 glucuronide |
|   |   | Oxymorphone[a] | 6 hydroxy-oxymorphone |
|   |   | Tapentadol | Tapentadol O-glucuronide |

*Abbreviation:* UGT, uridine diphosphate glucuronosyltransferase.
[a] Pharmacokinetics have not been studied in the elderly.
*Data from* McLachlan AJ, Bath S, Naganathan V, et al. Clinical pharmacology of analgesic medicines in older people: impact of frailty and cognitive impairment. Br J Clin Pharmacol 2011;71:351–64; and Smith HS. Opioid metabolism. Mayo Clin Proc 2009;84:613–24.

During phase II hepatic metabolism, medications have an additional molecule attached to facilitate excretion. For opioids, phase II metabolism by the isoenzyme uridine diphosphate glucuronosyltransferase is generally thought to be unaffected by age.[26–28] Again, the exception is morphine, because age-related reductions in hepatic blood flow lead to decreased clearance and increased half-life of high hepatic extraction drugs.[17]

The kidneys are involved in the elimination of all opioids. Furthermore, renal function, which can be estimated by glomerular filtration rate, is reduced with age.[18] Codeine, hydromorphone, meperidine, morphine, oxycodone, and tramadol all have renally cleared, active metabolites (see **Table 1**). Consequently, age-related decreases in renal function can lead to opioid toxicity with these opioids owing to the accumulation of active metabolic byproducts. Specifically, meperidine should be avoided in older adults because accumulation of its active metabolite (normeperidine) can cause neurotoxicity.[29] Only tramadol has specific dosing guidelines in those with a decreased glomerular filtration rate.[29]

In addition to the pharmacokinetic changes, it is important to emphasize that among older adults, enhanced pharmacodynamic sensitivity (ie, more pronounced effects at equivalent doses used in younger adults) is seen with all opioids.[19,22] Indeed, pharmacodynamic sensitivity helps to explain the risks of opioids unique to geriatric patients.[6,8,19,29,30] In a metaanalysis of pooled data from 6 observational studies, older adults exposed to opioids had a 38% increased likelihood of fractures (relative risk, 1.38; 95% CI, 1.15-1.66).[31] Moreover, the timing of opioid initiation may be an important consideration. Compared with new users of nonsteroidal anti-inflammatory drugs, individuals initiating opioid therapy for arthritis were 4 to 5 times more likely to have a fracture.[32–34]

Additionally, there is a dose–response relationship between opioid exposure and risk.[32,35] One study of 2341 older adults found that individuals taking 50 or more oral morphine equivalents (OME) daily had a 2-fold increased risk of fractures (adjusted hazard ratio, 2.00; 95% CI, 1.24–3.24).[35] However, this increased risk is not confined to opioids in isolation. Coadministration of opioids and other agents that affect the central nervous system (benzodiazepine receptor agonists, antipsychotics, tricyclic antidepressants, and selective serotonin reuptake inhibitors) has also been associated with falls and fractures.[36,37] As such, the administration of 3 or more central nervous system agents is now considered a clinically important drug–drug interaction in the 2015 American Geriatrics Society Beers Criteria, an explicit measure of potentially inappropriate prescribing in older adults.[29]

The link between opioids (alone and in combination with other medications affecting the central nervous system) and cognitive decline in older adults is well-established.[38] Moreover, a recent metaanalysis showed that opioids also increase the risk of delirium.[39] Meperidine was associated with the greatest risk of delirium, which is not surprising given its renally cleared neurotoxic metabolite. As such, its use in individuals with cognitive impairment or previous delirium is considered a drug–disease interaction per the 2015 American Geriatrics Society Beers Criteria.[29] It is important to note, however, that at least in 1 study of older adults hospitalized for hip fracture and who underwent surgical repair, the risk of delirium was inversely associated with opioid dose (**Fig. 1**).[40] Lower doses of opioids resulted in greater episodes of delirium, suggesting that undertreating severe pain is a greater risk factor for delirium than the drugs themselves. Again, meperidine was the most problematic, because individuals receiving this medication were more than 2 times as likely to develop delirium as those receiving other opioids.[40]

The incidence of many stereotypical adverse drug reactions associated with opioids, such as constipation, do not differ between younger and older adults.[6] All patients chronically taking regularly scheduled opioid analgesics may benefit from taking daily stimulant laxative (eg, bisacodyl, senna) to avoid constipation. Additional common symptoms such as nausea and dizziness often subside after a few days of therapy.[12] A recent study also found that individuals exposed to tramadol had more

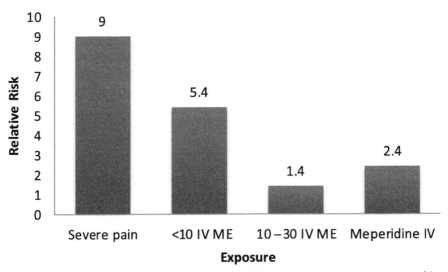

**Fig. 1.** Adjusted relative risk ratios for incident delirium. IV, intravenous; ME, morphine equivalents. (*Data from* Morrison RS, Magaziner J, Gilbert M, et al. Relationship between pain and opioid analgesics on the development of delirium following hip fracture. J Gerontol A Biol Sci Med Sci 2003;58:76–81.)

than a 2-fold increased risk of hospitalization for hypoglycemia (95% CI, 1.61–4.23) in the first 30 days after initiation compared with codeine.[41] Moreover, tramadol may exacerbate seizures in those with known epilepsy.[29] Other adverse drug events associated with opioid use specific to older adults are highlighted in **Fig. 2**.

Older individuals often take multiple medications (ie, polypharmacy), which increases their risk for adverse events stemming from drug–drug interactions involving opioids.[46,47] Because tramadol, meperidine, and fentanyl can increase serotonin levels, case reports suggest that they may precipitate serotonin syndrome when given with other medications (eg, selective serotonin reuptake inhibitors) that modulate the serotonin pathway.[48] Additionally, methadone has a known risk for torsades de pointes, and is especially problematic when given with other medications that increase the QT interval and/or inhibit CYP3A4 (eg, certain macrolide antibiotics).[49]

There is concern that the rapid increase in the use of opioids to treat CNCP in older adults may lead to abuse and misuse of this analgesic class. However, a recent review assessing the prevalence of opioid misuse in older adults estimated that 1% to 3% of older adults used opioids inappropriately, which was consistently less than the proportion of their younger counterparts.[12] Another study using data from the Researched Abuse, Diversion and Addiction-Related Surveillance System Poison Center Program evaluated 184,136 calls regarding opioid abuse (intentional incorrect use for the purposes of achieving a psychotropic effect), misuse (intentional incorrect use for reasons other than to achieve a psychotropic effect or suicidal intent), and suicidal intent.[50] Compared with controls aged 20 to 59, adults 60 years or older had a lower average annual rate of calls and lower proportion of calls for abuse, but a greater proportion of calls as misuse.[50] Furthermore, death from opioid overdose is less prevalent in those 65 years or older when compared with younger adults. In 2011, for example, 1.3 opioid-related deaths were seen per 100,000 adults 65 years or older, compared with 6.3 to 11.2 deaths per 100,000 adults of younger age groups.[51]

## OPTIMIZING OPIOIDS IN OLDER PERSONS

When nonpharmacologic modalities and nonopioid analgesics do not provide adequate relief for moderate-to-severe CNCP, opioids should be considered as adjunctive therapy. However, balancing potential risks and benefits associated with

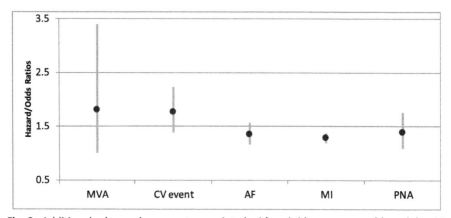

**Fig. 2.** Additional adverse drug events associated with opioid use among older adults. AF, atrial fibrillation; CV, cardiovascular event; MI, myocardial infarction; MVA, motor vehicle accident; PNA, pneumonia. (*Data from* Refs.[33,42–45])

opioids in older persons can be challenging. As such, we recommend the lowest tolerated dose that leads to acceptable relief of pain. **Table 2** provides a clinical algorithm for initiating and maintaining opioid dosage for severe pain. That these are suggestions only and that decisions should ultimately depend on severity of pain, functional status, expected duration that the pain will last, and patient preference. Nonetheless, the guidance outlined in **Table 2** regarding appropriate use for severe pain is based on the following principles.

1. Build a personal formulary and become comfortable with a few agents, rather than trying to learn caveats of the entire opioid cadre. We recommend prioritizing those opioids (tramadol, oxycodone, and morphine) in which pharmacokinetic, pharmacodynamic, and efficacy studies have been conducted in older persons.
2. Initiation phase doses of opioids should be lower than those used in a younger population, and subsequent titrations should be made slowly and under close supervision.
3. When initiating therapy in an opioid-naïve patient, avoid using long-acting opioids (methadone, levorphanol, fentanyl patch, or opioids delivered by extended-release dosage forms). In all situations, nonopioid analgesics (ie, acetaminophen) should be continued to facilitate "opioid-sparing" dosing.
4. Once a stable daily dose is established, consider changing therapy during the maintenance phase to sustained release opioids on a regularly scheduled basis in cases of severe pain, with immediate release opioids prescribed as needed for

**Table 2**
**Initial and maintenance opioid therapy for severe chronic noncancer pain in older adults**

| Dosing Option | Initiation Phase | Maintenance Phase |
|---|---|---|
| 1 | Tramadol IR 50 mg ½ tablet 1–2 times daily AND Tramadol IR ½ tablet every 6 h as needed[b] *When >200 mg tramadol is required for analgesia, convert to maintenance phase.* | Morphine SR[a] or oxycodone SR every 12 h AND Morphine IR or oxycodone IR every 6 h as needed |
| 2 | Oxycodone IR 5 mg ½ - 1 tablet every 6 h AND Oxycodone IR ½ tablet every 3 h as needed[b] | Oxycodone SR 1 tablet every 12 h AND Oxycodone IR 1 tablet every 6 h as needed |
| 3 | Morphine solution[c] 2.5–5 mg every 6 h AND Morphine solution 2.5 mg every 3 h as needed | Morphine SR[a] 1 tablet every 12 h AND Morphine IR 1 tablet every 6 h as needed |

*Abbreviations:* IR, immediate release; SR, sustained release.
  [a] Special cases: patients with a "true allergy" to codeine/morphine class drugs may consider fentanyl patch (12 μg is approximately equal to 30 mg oral morphine equivalents).
  [b] Every 3 to 7 days, may increase daily dosage of tramadol by 25 mg, oxycodone by 5 mg and morphine by 2.5 mg.
  [c] For those with swallowing difficulties.
*Data from* Refs.[18,19,29]

breakthrough pain. To convert from oxycodone immediate release to sustained release, simply add up the total daily dose of immediate release medication, and then administer one-half of the total amount every 12 hours. When switching from morphine immediate release to sustained release, give the full daily dose every 24 hours or one-half the daily dose every 12 hours, depending on the least expensive formulation available.

5. Cross-tolerance must be taken into consideration when switching opioids. The conversion factor 50 mg tramadol = 10 mg oxycodone = 10 mg OME may be used to convert between opioids. Lower the daily dose of the newly prescribed opioid by 25 to 50% OME. For example, when converting from tramadol 200 mg daily to oral morphine, 200 mg = 40 OME. The appropriate dose of morphine sustained release is 10 mg every 12 hours, and then 5 mg of immediate release every 6 hours as needed for breakthrough pain.

6. Pharmacists and palliative care/pain experts are available to provide consults for challenging cases, including those requiring large doses of opioids ($\geq$100–120 OME daily).

## SUMMARY

There are important age-related changes in the pharmacokinetics/pharmacodynamics of opioids. Thus to minimize adverse drug events, opioids should be reserved for moderate/severe CNCP not responsive to other treatment modalities and starting doses should be low and changes in doses should be made slowly.

## REFERENCES

1. American Geriatrics Society Panel on the Pharmacological Management of Persistent Pain in Older Persons. Pharmacological management of persistent pain in older persons. J Am Geriatr Soc 2009;57:1331–46.
2. Abdulla A, Adams N, Bone M, et al. British Geriatric Society Guidance on the management of pain in older people. Age Ageing 2013;42:i1–57.
3. The medical letter: drugs for pain. Treat Guidel Med Lett 2013;11(128):31–42.
4. American Society of Health System Pharmacists. 2011 update to demystifying opioid conversion calculations: a guide for effective dosing. Available at: http://www.ashp.org/doclibrary/bookstore/p1985/2011-update.aspx. Accessed January 7, 2016.
5. Pharmacist's Letter 2012. Equianalgesic dosing of opioids for pain management. Available at: http://prescribersletter.therapeuticresearch.com/pl/ArticlePDF.aspx?cs=&s=PRL&DocumentFileID=0&DetailID=280821&SegmentID=0. Accessed January 7, 2016.
6. Campbell CI, Weisner C, Leresche L, et al. Age and gender trends in long-term opioid analgesic use for noncancer pain. Am J Public Health 2010;100:2541–7.
7. Marcum ZA, Perera S, Donohue JM, et al. Analgesic use for knee and hip osteoarthritis in community-dwelling elders. Pain Med 2011;12:1628–36.
8. Karp JF, Lee CW, McGovern J, et al. Clinical and demographic covariates of chronic opioid and non-opioid analgesic use in rural-dwelling older adults: the MoVIES project. Int Psychogeriatr 2013;25:1801–10.
9. Steinman MA, Komaiko KD, Fung KZ, et al. Use of opioids and other analgesics by older adults in the United States, 1999-2010. Pain Med 2015;16:319–27.
10. Lapane KL, Quilliam BJ, Chow W, et al. Pharmacologic management of noncancer pain among nursing home residents. J Pain Symptom Manage 2013;45:33–42.

11. Veal FC, Bereznicki LR, Thompson AJ, et al. Use of opioid analgesics in older Australian. Pain Med 2015;16:1519–27.

12. Papaleontiou M, Henderson CR Jr, Turner BJ, et al. Outcomes associated with opioid use in the treatment of chronic noncancer pain in older adults: a systematic review and meta-analysis. J Am Geriatr Soc 2010;58:1353–69.

13. Chou R, Turner JA, Devine EB, et al. The effectiveness and risks of long-term opioid therapy for chronic pain: a systematic review for a National Institutes of Health Pathways to Prevention Workshop. Ann Intern Med 2015;162:276.

14. Eriksen J, Sjøgren P, Bruera E, et al. Critical issues on opioids in chronic noncancer pain: an epidemiological study. Pain 2006;125:172–9.

15. Roy S, Flynn G. Transdermal delivery of narcotic analgesics: pH, anatomical, and subject influences on cutaneous permeability of fentanyl and sufentanil. Pharm Res 1990;7:842–7.

16. Al-Tawil N, Odar-Cederlöf I, Berggren AC, et al. Pharmacokinetics of transdermal buprenorphine patch in the elderly. Eur J Clin Pharmacol 2013;69:143–9.

17. Baillie SP, Bateman DN, Coates PE, et al. Age and the pharmacokinetics of morphine. Age Ageing 1989;18:258–62.

18. Hanlon JT, Guary DR, Ives TJ. Oral analgesics: efficacy, mechanism of action, pharmacokinetics, adverse effects, drug interactions, and practical recommendations for use in older adults. In: Gibson SJ, Weiner DK, editors. Pain in older persons. Progress in Pain Research and Management. IIASP Press; 2005. p. 205–22.

19. McLachlan AJ, Bath S, Naganathan V, et al. Clinical pharmacology of analgesic medicines in older people: impact of frailty and cognitive impairment. Br J Clin Pharmacol 2011;71:351–64.

20. Liukas A, Kuusniemi K, Aantaa R, et al. Plasma concentrations of oral oxycodone are greatly increased in the elderly. Clin Pharmacol Ther 2008;84:462–7.

21. Saari TI, Ihmsen H, Neuvonen PJ, et al. Oxycodone clearance is markedly reduced with advancing age: a population pharmacokinetic study. Br J Anaesth 2012;108:491–8.

22. Scott JC, Stanski DR. Decreased fentanyl and alfentanil dose requirements with age. A simultaneous pharmacokinetic and pharmacodynamic evaluation. J Pharmacol Exp Ther 1987;240:159–66.

23. Hanlon JT, Weiner D. Methadone for chronic pain in older adults: blast from the past but are we ready for it to return to prime time? Pain Med 2009;10:287–8.

24. Likar R, Wittels M, Molnar M, et al. Pharmacokinetic and pharmacodynamic properties of tramadol IR and SR in elderly patients: a prospective, age-group-controlled study. Clin Ther 2006;28:2022–39.

25. Somogyi AA, Coller JK, Barratt DT. Pharmacogenetics of opioid response. Clin Pharmacol Ther 2015;97:125–7.

26. Durnin C, Hind ID, Ghani SP, et al. Pharmacokinetics of oral immediate-release hydromorphone (Dilaudid IR) in young and elderly subjects. Proc West Pharmacol Soc 2001;44:79–80.

27. Smit JW, Häufel T, Ravenstijn P, et al. Pharmacokinetics of tapentadol in healthy elderly and young subjects. J Clin Pharmacol 2010;50:1079.

28. King S, Forbes K, Hanks GW, et al. A systematic review of the use of opioid medication for those with moderate to severe cancer pain and renal impairment: a European Palliative Care Research Collaborative opioid guidelines project. Palliat Med 2011;25:525–32.

29. By the American Geriatrics Society 2015 Beers Criteria Update Expert Panel. American Geriatrics Society 2015 updated beers criteria for potentially inappropriate medication use in older adults. J Am Geriatr Soc 2015;63:2227–46.

30. Huang AR, Mallet L. Prescribing opioids in older people. Maturitas 2013;74: 123–9.

31. Takkouche B, Montes-Martínez A, Gill SS, et al. Psychotropic medications and the risk of fracture: a meta-analysis. Drug Saf 2007;30:171–84.

32. Miller M, Stürmer T, Azrael D, et al. Opioid analgesics and the risk of fractures in older adults with arthritis. J Am Geriatr Soc 2011;59:430–8.

33. Solomon DH, Rassen JA, Glynn RJ, et al. The comparative safety of opioids for nonmalignant pain in older adults. Arch Intern Med 2010;170:1979–86.

34. Rolita L, Spegman A, Tang X, et al. Greater number of narcotic analgesic prescriptions for osteoarthritis is associated with falls and fractures in elderly adults. J Am Geriatr Soc 2013;61:335–40.

35. Saunders KW, Dunn KM, Merrill JO, et al. Relationship of opioid use and dosage levels to fractures in older chronic pain patients. J Gen Intern Med 2010;25: 310–5.

36. Boudreau RM, Hanlon JT, Roumani YF, et al. Central nervous system medication use and incident mobility limitation in community elders: the Health, Aging, and Body Composition study. Pharmacoepidemiol Drug Saf 2009;18:916–22.

37. Hanlon JT, Boudreau RM, Roumani YF, et al. Number and dosage of central nervous system medications on recurrent falls in community elders: the Health, Aging and Body Composition study. J Gerontol A Biol Sci Med Sci 2009;64A:492–8.

38. Puustinen J, Nurminen J, Löppönen M, et al. Use of CNS medications and cognitive decline in the aged: a longitudinal population-based study. BMC Geriatr 2011;11:70.

39. Clegg A, Young JB. Which medications to avoid in people at risk of delirium: a systematic review. Age Ageing 2011;40:23–9.

40. Morrison RS, Magaziner J, Gilbert M, et al. Relationship between pain and opioid analgesics on the development of delirium following hip fracture. J Gerontol A Biol Sci Med Sci 2003;58:76–81.

41. Fournier JP, Azoulay L, Yin H, et al. Tramadol use and the risk of hospitalization for hypoglycemia in patients with noncancer pain. JAMA Intern Med 2015;175: 186–93.

42. Leveille SG, Buchner DM, Koepsell TD, et al. Psychoactive medications and injurious motor vehicle collisions involving older drivers. Epidemiology 1994;5:591–8.

43. Qureshi WT, O'Neal WT, Khodneva Y, et al. Association between opioid use and atrial fibrillation: the Reasons for Geographic and Racial Differences in Stroke (REGARDS) study. JAMA Intern Med 2015;175:1058–60.

44. Li L, Setoguchi S, Cabral H, et al. Opioid use for noncancer pain and risk of myocardial infarction amongst adults. J Intern Med 2013;273:511–26.

45. Dublin S, Walker RL, Jackson ML, et al. Use of opioids or benzodiazepines and risk of pneumonia in older adults: a population-based case-control study. J Am Geriatr Soc 2011;59:1899–907.

46. Budnitz DS, Lovegrove MC, Shehab N, et al. Emergency hospitalizations for adverse drug events in older Americans. N Engl J Med 2011;365:2002–12.

47. Richarz U, Jacobs A, Spina E. How frequently are contraindicated or warned against combinations of drugs prescribed to patients receiving long-term opioid therapy for chronic pain? Pharmacoepidemiol Drug Saf 2012;21:453–62.

48. Hanlon JT, Wang X, Castle NG, et al. Potential underuse, overuse and inappropriate use of antidepressants in older veteran nursing home patients. J Am Geriatr Soc 2011;59:1412–20.
49. Ray WA, Chung CP, Murray KT, et al. Out-of-hospital mortality among patients receiving methadone for noncancer pain. JAMA Intern Med 2015;175:420–7.
50. West NA, Severtson SG, Green JL, et al. Trends in abuse and misuse of prescription opioids among older adults. Drug Alcohol Depend 2015;149:117–21.
51. Chen LH, Hedegaard H, Warner M. Drug-poisoning deaths involving opioid analgesics: United States, 1999–2011. NCHS Data Brief 2014;166:1–8. Available at: http://www.cdc.gov/nchs/data/databriefs/db166.pdf. Accessed January 7, 2016.

# Exercise and Movement-based Therapies in Geriatric Pain Management

Sean Laubenstein, DPT[a], Katherine Beissner, PT, PhD[b],*

## KEYWORDS

- Exercise • Tai chi • Movement therapy • Endurance • Strength • Pain

## KEY POINTS

- Pain is frequently seen as a barrier to initiating and sustaining exercise, but exercise is still recommended by expert panels as an important part of a comprehensive pain management program.
- Most research on exercise in older adults with pain problems has focused on resistance and aerobic exercise, and both seem to be effective in enhancing function.
- Exercise must be done at an appropriate frequency, intensity, and duration in order to achieve optimal effects, but individual differences make routine prescription difficult and a tailored approach is likely to enhance adherence.

## INTRODUCTION

Although pain is often identified as a reason to limit movement,[1] exercise is widely recognized as an effective method of managing pain in older adults.[2–5] Several organizations and panels have provided consensus documents, guidelines, and suggestions for exercise prescription in older adults,[2,5,6] some organized around a particular type of exercise (eg, resistance or aerobics) and others setting parameters for individuals with a specific diagnosis.

Despite its clinically established role in pain control, the mechanisms by which exercise modulates pain are not well understood. Recent review articles indicate that in healthy people there is evidence of exercise-induced analgesia through release of endogenous opioids.[7] However, this is not well studied in adults with pain problems, and there is some evidence that the mechanism may differ in individuals with chronic pain.[7,8]

Disclosures: The authors have nothing to disclose.
[a] Chittenango Physical Therapy, Chittenango, NY, USA; [b] Department of Physical Therapy Education, SUNY Upstate Medical University, 750 East Adams Street, Syracuse, NY 13210, USA
* Corresponding author.
*E-mail address:* beissnek@upstate.edu

Clin Geriatr Med 32 (2016) 737–762
http://dx.doi.org/10.1016/j.cger.2016.06.002
0749-0690/16/© 2016 Elsevier Inc. All rights reserved.

geriatric.theclinics.com

A review article by Beckwee and colleagues[9] describes 5 potential pain reduction mechanisms applicable to patients with osteoarthritis (OA), with considerable overlap between categories. A neuromuscular impact on pain is related to decreased joint loading through improved motor control, increased joint stability, and increased energy absorption capacity of muscles.[9] The impact of exercise on periarticular structures may reduce pain through improved flexibility, enhanced density and quality of the connective tissues, and a potential impact on bony mass.[9] The speculated intra-articular benefits of exercise include improved cartilage structure, reduced inflammation (related to decreased compressive forces), and improved joint nutrition.[9] General fitness benefits that may decrease pain include a reduction in comorbidities; weight loss leading to decreased joint loading; and improved aerobic fitness, which enhances well-being.[9] In addition, the psychosocial impact of exercise is speculated to decrease pain through reduction in depressive symptoms, improved affect attributed to generally enhanced well-being, a placebo effect, and improved self-efficacy.[9] The investigators surmise that a combination of benefits from each category is responsible for the pain-reducing effects of physical exercise.

This article reviews available literature regarding the efficacy of movement-based therapies for pain management in adults aged 60 years and older. Studies were selected from a search of the PubMed and CINAHL (Cumulative Index to Nursing and Allied Health Literature) online databases. **Box 1** shows the search strings used and the characteristics of each search. In addition to these searches, a manual search of the reference lists included in pertinent systematic reviews was conducted. Studies included in this review enrolled adults aged 60 years and older with a pain-related disorder, use at least 1 pain-related outcome measure, were published after 1995, and incorporated a movement-based therapy as a main intervention. To focus on the impact of exercise on older adults, studies enrolling both younger and older subjects were only included if the data were analyzed and reported separately for the older group. Case reports were excluded. Thirty-four studies met inclusion criteria. Exercise programs included in this review were delivered in a variety of venues, including community centers (such as senior centers), physical therapy clinics, and the home environment. Combinations of these venues were also seen, with some programs beginning in community settings but transitioning to increasing levels of independence for long-term continuation of exercise.

This article is organized by exercise type, and each section includes a summary of the literature and interpretation of the evidence. Although the primary focus is exercise for pain management among older adults, functional outcomes were also assessed in most of the studies reviewed. **Box 2** shows the commonly used outcome measures

---

**Box 1**
**Search characteristics**

| Database | PubMed | CINAHL |
|---|---|---|
| Search String | ((((("Exercise"[Majr]) OR "Exercise Therapy"[Majr]) OR "Exercise Movement Techniques"[Majr])) AND (("Pain"[Majr]) OR "Pain Management"[Majr]))) AND (("Aged"[Mesh]) OR "Aged, 80 and over"[Mesh]) | (MM "Exercise+") OR (MM "Therapeutic Exercise+") OR (MM "Dance Therapy") OR (MM "Tai Chi") OR (MM "Yoga") AND (MM "Pain+") AND (MH "Aged+") PubMed results were excluded as duplicates |
| Number of Results | 537 | 107 |

| Box 2 | |
|---|---|
| **Commonly used outcome measures** | |
| **Measure** | **Abbreviation** |
| Pain Intensity | |
| Numerical Rating Scale | NRS |
| Visual Analog Scale | VAS |
| Physical Performance Measures | |
| 30-Second Chair Rise | — |
| Gait Speed | — |
| Six-minute Walk Test | 6MWT |
| Timed Up and Go | TUG |
| Self-report | |
| Arthritis Impact Measurement Scales 2 | AIMS 2 |
| Arthritis Self-efficacy Scale | ASES |
| Elderly Mobility Scale | EMS |
| Fear Avoidance Beliefs Questionnaire | FABQ |
| Neck Disability Index | NDI |
| Oswestry Disability Questionnaire | OSQ |
| Pain Self-efficacy Questionnaire | PSEQ |
| Quality of Life Questionnaires | QUALEFFO |
| Roland Morris Disability Questionnaire | RMDQ |
| Short Form 36 | SF36 |
| The Western Ontario and McMaster Universities Arthritis Index | WOMAC |

and their abbreviations. Most of the studies commented only on statistical significance, but we were concerned with the clinical significance of results. For commonly used outcome measures, established values were used for minimal detectable change (MDC) or the minimal clinically important difference (MCID) to interpret results.

## RESISTANCE EXERCISE

Resistance exercise involves the use of an external force to resist a body movement, with the goal of increasing muscle strength and muscle power.[6] Guidelines for resistance exercise have been specified by the American College of Sports Medicine (ACSM) and the American Geriatrics Society (AGS), as summarized in **Box 3**.

Seven studies examined the impact of resistance exercise on pain and function, most focused on strength around the knee. Facility-based group resistance training was the most prevalent method used, with progression of the program incorporated into most studies by increasing resistance, sets, repetitions, and/or duration. **Table 1** summarizes the literature on resistance exercise.

A variety of forms of resistance training were examined. Two studies used body-weight resistance,[10,11] and another used a combination of body-weight and elastic-band exercises.[12] Using weights to progress treatment allows greater precision in the progression of exercise, which is often based on a percentage of the 1-repetition maximum (1RM; the maximum weight that can be moved through a range of motion only 1 time). Three studies used weights for resistance.[13–15] Another study examined the impact of physical therapist–provided strengthening exercises plus conventional treatment (defined as heat and electrotherapy), but did not specify the mode of resistance used.[16]

Collectively, these trials suggest that resistance training constitutes a safe and effective way to reduce pain and improve function in older adults with pain. Two trials

| | | |
|---|---|---|
| **Box 3** | | |
| **Resistance exercise guidelines** | | |
| **Parameters** | **ACSM Older Adult/Adult Recommendations**[6] | **AGS Older Adults with Osteoarthritis Pain Recommendations**[2] |
| Frequency | 2–3 sessions per week for each major muscle group | • Isometric: can be performed daily<br>• Isotonic 2–3 sessions weekly |
| Intensity | • 40%–50% 1RM in older adults initiating exercise<br>• 60%–70% 1RM in experienced exercisers<br>• 20%–50% 1RM to train power in older adults<br>• <50% to train muscular endurance | • Isometric: 40%–60% maximum voluntary contraction (low to moderate intensity)<br>• Isotonic: low resistance (40% 1RM) to high resistance (60% 1RM), with a maximum of 80% 1RM |
| Repetitions | • 10–15 repetitions for older adults beginning a program to build strength<br>• 8–12 repetitions for most adults to train power and strength<br>• 15–20 repetitions to build muscular endurance | • Isometric: hold each contraction for 1–6 s<br>• Isotonic: 6–15 repetitions |
| Sets | • 1 set can be sufficient in older adults<br>• 2–4 sets can be used to increase strength and power<br>• 2 or fewer sets should be used in muscular endurance exercises | • Isometric: 1–10 submaximal contractions per key muscle group<br>• Isometric: 1 set |
| Type | • Multijoint exercises should be prioritized more than single joint<br>• Appropriate resistance may be provided by machines, weights, bands, body weight, and so forth | Not specified |
| Pattern | • 2–3 min of rest between sets of repetitions<br>• At least 48 h between sessions for each muscle group | Not specified |
| Progression | • Progression should be gradual and can come from:<br>  ○ Increased resistance<br>  ○ More repetitions<br>  ○ Increased frequency of exercise | Not specified |
| *Abbreviations:* OA, osteoarthritis; 1RM, 1-repetition maximum. | | |

reported a small number of adverse outcomes and all trials showed improvements in pain and/or function postintervention. However, the magnitude of the improvements reported is questionable because few studies reported on the clinical significance of their findings, and our analysis revealed that most statistical improvements did not exceed the MDC or MCID for the outcome. Note that details on the intensity of exercise were not specified in all studies, and when details were provided the intensity was generally low and varied. Low-intensity exercise is unlikely to optimize exercise outcomes. For effective strengthening, muscles must be pushed to the point of overload. The ACSM guidelines specify 40% to 50% of 1RM as the minimal stimulus for

**Table 1**
Resistance exercise studies

| Study | Participants | Interventions | Outcome Measures | Setting and Duration | Major Results |
|---|---|---|---|---|---|
| Ettinger et al,[13] 1997, RCT | 439 community-dwelling adults aged ≥60 y with knee OA | Aerobic group: walking program at 50%–70% of HRR Resistance group: weight training for LE and UE Control group: health education | Self-reported disability test, physical performance test, knee pain with activity questionnaire | Group exercise at a facility for 3 mo, home-based program for the following 15 mo | Aerobic and resistance groups reported significantly less physical disability than the control; both intervention groups reported significantly less pain than the control group; aerobic group improved significantly more on all (and the resistance group improved more on most) physical performance tests than the control; resistance group compliance was 78%, aerobic group compliance was 68% |
| Hasegawa et al,[11] 2013, non-RCT | 320 adults aged ≥65 y at risk for requiring long-term care; most participants (n = 252) reported chronic knee or low back pain | Intervention group: resistance training for legs, core, and back using body weight; lecture on pain management and exercise Control group: observed for 12 wk | VAS, RMDQ, WOMAC, TUG, 5-min Walk Test, SLS | Community-based group exercise for 12 wk with an HEP | VAS improved more than the MCID for men and women in the intervention group. Women improved significantly more than the control on all physical performance measures, WOMAC score, and VAS pain |

(continued on next page)

**Table 1**
*(continued)*

| Study | Participants | Interventions | Outcome Measures | Setting and Duration | Major Results |
|---|---|---|---|---|---|
| Lim et al,[16] 2013, single-group repeated measures | 12 adults aged ≥65 y with diagnosed knee OA | Intervention group: hot pack and electrotherapy followed by 40 min of PT-supervised exercise including resistance training | VAS | Clinic based for 10 wk | VAS scores decreased significantly from baseline in participants |
| Liu-Ambrose et al,[14] 2005, RCT | 98 nonexercising white women aged 75–85 y with diagnosis of osteoporosis or osteopenia | Resistance group: free-weight training for UEs, LEs, and trunk at 50%–60% 1RM progressing to 75%–85% 1RM. Agility group: dance moves, obstacle courses, ball games. Control group: stretching and relaxation exercises | ODQ, QUALEFFO | Facility-based group exercise for 25 wk | All 3 groups improved on the ODQ with no between-group differences. Resistance and agility groups showed improvement in QUALEFFO score with no between-group differences. Compliance was 85% in the resistance group |
| Murphy et al,[15] 2008, RCT | 54 adults with hip or knee OA with a mean age of 75 y | Intervention group: PREs plus education on symptom management and activity training eg, (body mechanics, activity pacing). Control group: PREs plus Arthritis Foundation information–based health education | WOMAC, Arthritis Self-efficacy Scale, 6MWT, TUG, self-reported and objective physical activity | Facility-based group exercise for 4 wk, followed by an HEP for 2 mo | There were no significant between-group differences, except in objective physical activity, favoring the intervention group with a small to moderate effect size; WOMAC pain subscale scores decreased in both groups |

| | | | | | |
|---|---|---|---|---|---|
| Petrella et al,[10] 2000, RCT | 177 adults aged ≥65 y with OA pain in at least 1 knee | Intervention group: progressive exercise program for the LEs using household items and body weight. ROM exercises were also included. Control group: stretching and LE joint unloading (both groups received oxaprozin 1200 mg daily) | WOMAC, VAS, self-paced walking, self-paced stepping | Home-based program for 8 wk | WOMAC pain subscale improved more than the MDC in both groups; intervention group also improved more than the MDC for WOMAC physical performance; VAS scores decreased more than the MCID in the intervention group; intervention group improved significantly more than the control group on physical performance measures and WOMAC pain and disability scores |
| Wong et al,[12] 2005, pretest, posttest | 22 adults aged ≥60 y with knee pain on most days | Intervention group: a weekly exercise class and education provided at a facility by a PT via videoconference. Exercises included functional and elastic band resistance exercises. An HEP was provided | SF-36, TUG, WOMAC | Facility-based with concurrent HEP for 12 wk | Significant improvement in all WOMAC subscales. Significant improvement in TUG scores |

*Abbreviations:* HEP, home exercise program; HRR, heart rate reserve; LE, lower extremity; MCID, minimal clinically important difference; 6MWT, Six-minute Walk Test; OA, osteoarthritis; ODQ, oswestry disability questionnaire; PRE, progressive resistance exercise; PT, physical therapist; QUALEFFO, Quality of Life Questionnaires; RCT, randomized controlled trial; RMDQ, Roland Morris Disability Questionnaire; ROM, range of motion; SF-36, Short Form-36; SLS, single leg stance; TUG, Timed Up and Go; UE, upper extremity; VAS, Visual Analog Scale; WOMAC, Western Ontario and McMaster Universities Arthritis Index.
*Data from* Refs.[10–16]

**Table 2**
Aerobic exercise

| Study | Participants | Interventions | Outcome Measures | Setting and Duration | Major Results |
|---|---|---|---|---|---|
| Ettinger et al,[13] 1997, RCT | 439 community-dwelling adults aged ≥60 y with knee OA | Aerobic group: supervised walking at 50%–70% of heart rate reserve (HRR) Resistance group: weight training Control group: health education | Self-reported disability; physical performance test; knee pain with activity questionnaire | Group exercise at facility for 3 mo, home program for 15 mo | Aerobic and resistance groups reported significantly less physical disability than the control group; both intervention groups reported significantly less pain than the control group. The aerobic group improved significantly more on all (and the resistance group improved more on most) physical performance tests than the control; resistance group compliance was 78%, aerobic group compliance was 68% |
| Ferrell et al,[21] 1997, RCT | 29 ambulatory veterans aged ≥65 y with chronic LE or back pain | Group 1: supervised and monitored fitness walking Group 2: pain self-management education with weekly phone follow-up Group 3: printed pain management educational materials | NRS; Patient Pain Questionnaire; SF-36; 6MWT; 30-s chair rise | Group 1: facility-based program for 6 wk | Fitness walking group improved in pain intensity, SF-36, 6MWT, 30-s chair rise; pain self-management group showed improved pain knowledge and 30-s chair rise |

| Study | Population | Intervention | Outcome Measures | Setting | Results |
|---|---|---|---|---|---|
| Nyrop et al,[18] 2014, pretest-posttest | 19 female breast cancer survivors aged ≥65 y receiving aromatase inhibitor therapy, with self-diagnosed arthritis or joint pain; participants able to ambulate and tolerate moderate physical activity | Walk With Ease: self-directed walking program | VAS for pain, stiffness, fatigue; Arthritis Self-efficacy Scale | Home-based 6-wk program | Significant improvement in joint stiffness (effect size 0.56); no improvement in pain, fatigue, or self-efficacy |
| Rhudy et al,[20] 2007, RCT | 212 community-dwelling adults aged 60-80 y receiving treatment at a VA facility | Individualized walking program established with nurse. Group 1, 20 personal phone calls over 12 mo; group 2, 10 personal and 10 automated phone calls; group 3, no phone calls | SF-36, bodily pain item; pain frequency; self-reported walking for exercise | Home-based with follow-up at 6 and 12 mo | Improvement in time spent walking for all groups; no change in pain intensity or frequency; pain was not a barrier to initiating or maintaining walking |
| Talbot et al,[19] 2003, RCT | 34 community-dwelling adults aged ≥60 y with knee pain and diagnosis of OA | Education: arthritis self-management program. Walk+: arthritis self-management and pedometer-based walking program with nurse-led education/goal setting | Present Pain Intensity Scale; Pain Rating Index - Total; walking speed, timed 3× chair rise; timed stair climb; daily steps walked; strength | Home-based exercise for 12 wk with 12-wk follow-up | Improved daily steps walked and speed of walking in Walk+ group. No change in pain measures, stair climb, or chair rise for either group. Performance deteriorated by 3-mo follow-up |

*Abbreviations:* NRS, Numerical Rating Scale; VA, Veterans' Affairs.
*Data from* Refs.[13,18–21]

deconditioned older adults beginning a strengthening program, and 60% to 70% of 1RM for more experienced exercisers.[6] A consensus document published by the AGS[2] is largely in agreement with the ACSM's recommendations.

Progression is another key element of effective resistance training. Progressive resistance exercise (PRE) ensures that muscles are continually overloaded, providing the requisite stimulus for strengthening.[17] The progression scheme followed by some of the reviewed studies is likely insufficient to yield continued overload. The trial conducted by Liu-Ambrose and colleagues[14] was the only study to explicitly follow ACSM recommendations. It is likely that insufficient resistance was provided in many of the reviewed studies, yielding minimal changes in pain and function.

## AEROBIC EXERCISE

Walking is the most common form of aerobic/endurance exercise advocated for older patients with pain. Because there are no equipment requirements (aside from supportive shoes) walking is accessible to most older adults with pain problems. Most of the research has focused on individualized walking programs, with various levels of education and support for beginning and adhering to a progressive program. This literature is summarized in **Table 2**.

Studies of walking programs were typically small and varied in terms of the level of support provided, including (1) a single instructional session,[18] (2) instruction plus regular review of progress,[19] (3) individualized program development with long-term follow-up,[20] (4) group-based walking program with progression of intensity,[21] and (5) a facility-based program that used exercise testing to prescribe intensity.[13]

The research has different levels of follow-up as well, either reporting outcomes at the end of the prescribed program[13,18,21] or examining longer-term impact.[19,20,22]

Guidelines for aerobic exercise are available from both ACSM and AGS (**Box 4**). Most of the research on aerobic exercise incorporated frequencies consistent with these guidelines, but the intensity of exercise was variable, and most often was not described. Differentiating between intensity levels may not be important for pain control, but likely affects aerobic conditioning.

In sum, these studies show that walking programs can benefit older adults with pain problems. Although there are differences with regard to the impact of such exercise programs on various pain measures, the improvement in function was consistent across studies. Although a comparison of effect sizes was not possible, it seems that supervised and monitored programs provide the most benefit. Adherence to exercise affects the gains achieved,[13] so interventions geared toward sustaining the walking program are important in maintaining long-term benefit.

## MULTIMODAL EXERCISE

The exercise guidelines recommended by ACSM and AGS include multiple types of exercise, including strength, aerobic conditioning, and stretching or balance training.[2,6] Most of the research examining the impact of multimodal exercise programs is based on group classes, with most including resistance and aerobic exercise. **Table 3** summarizes this literature.

Two standardized programs that are nationally available have reported outcomes for older patients with pain, including the 8-week Fit and Strong intervention[22,23] and the 6-session, weekly Arthritis Self-help Course.[24] Other group exercise programs were developed for research purposes, and varied in the degree of individualization, exercise progression, and class frequency.[11,25–27]

**Box 4**
**Aerobic exercise guidelines**

| Parameters | ACSM Older Adult/Adult Recommendations[6] | AGS Older Adults with OA Pain Recommendations[2] |
|---|---|---|
| Frequency | • 5 or more days per week of moderate exercise<br>Or<br>• 3 or more days per week of vigorous exercise<br>Or<br>• 3–5 d/wk of combined moderate and vigorous exercise | 3–5 d/wk |
| Intensity | • Moderate to vigorous intensity<br>• Light to moderate intensity for deconditioned adults | • 40%–60% of $Vo_{2max}$ or $HR_{max}$<br>• Low to moderate intensity<br>• RPE: 12–14 |
| Time | • 30–60 min of moderate-intensity exercise per day or 20–60 min of vigorous-intensity exercise per day<br>• Durations of <20 min can be beneficial in sedentary individuals beginning a program | 20–30 min/d of aerobic exercise |
| Type | Exercise involving major muscle groups that is continuous, rhythmic, regular, and purposeful | Not specified |
| Volume | • 500–1000 MET-min or more per week<br>• >7000 steps per day if walking is the mode of exercise | Not specified |
| Pattern | • Aerobic exercise may be performed in 1 bout, or intervals of $\geq$10 min to obtain the desired number of daily minutes<br>• Bouts of <10 min may be appropriate in severely deconditioned adults | Not specified |
| Progression | • Gradual progression provided by increasing:<br>  ○ Duration of the exercise<br>  ○ Frequency of the exercise<br>  ○ Intensity of the exercise | Not specified |

*Abbreviations:* $HR_{max}$, maximum heart rate; MET-min, metabolic equivalent per minute; RPE, rating of perceived exertion; $Vo_{2max}$, maximum oxygen uptake.

Combining multimodal exercise with other interventions may be important for certain populations. One study examined the addition of spinal manipulative therapy to exercise,[28] and another explored the impact of a diet plus exercise intervention for obese older adults with pain.[29]

The results of these studies are varied, and, in addition to the importance of exercise intensity (noted earlier), the frequency of exercise interventions also seems to affect the outcome. The 2 research programs that used group exercise 3 times a week resulted in meaningful changes in both pain and function,[22,23,29] but meaningful effects were not seen consistently in studies with a lower frequency of group exercise. Each of the programs that included group sessions 1 or 2 times per week included a home exercise program with written or compact disc–based instruction, but levels of

**Table 3**
Multimodal exercise

| Study | Participants | Interventions | Outcome Measures | Setting and Duration | Major Results |
|---|---|---|---|---|---|
| Hasegawa et al,[48] 2010, RCT | 28 older adults with knee joint pain | Intervention, weekly group exercise with warm-up, resistance, balance, and cool-down exercises + home program; control, no intervention | NRS, 30-s repeated chair rise; TUG | Community center; 12 wk | Intervention group had improved pain intensity, chair rise, and TUG; improvements in pain intensity and TUG were not clinically meaningful |
| Hughes et al,[23] 2004, RCT | 150 community-dwelling adults aged ≥60 y with physician-diagnosed LE OA | Intervention, Fit and Strong program with resistance training and fitness walking + 30-min group discussion; Control, educational booklet and community resource list | Arthritis Self-efficacy Scale, WOMAC, 5-repetition chair rise time, 6MWT | Community setting, 8 wk with home exercise thereafter. 6-mo postbaseline follow-up | Intervention group, meaningful improvement in WOMAC and 6MWT at 8 wk and sustained at 6 mo; control group had improved 6MWT at 8 wk and 6 mo; no between-group differences in pain self-efficacy |
| Hughes et al,[22] 2006, RCT | 225 community-dwelling adults aged ≥60 y with physician-diagnosed LE OA | Intervention, Fit and Strong program with resistance training and fitness walking + 30-min group discussion; control, educational booklet and community resource list | Arthritis Self-efficacy Scale, self-efficacy for exercise, WOMAC, Geri-AIMS Pain Scale, exercise adherence, 5-repetition chair rise, 6MWT | Community setting, 8 wk with home exercise thereafter. 6-mo and 12-mo postbaseline follow-up | Intervention group showed improved exercise adherence, self-efficacy for exercise WOMAC and 6MWT scores at 6 mo were sustained at 12 mo |

| Study | Population | Intervention | Outcome Measures | Setting/Duration | Results |
|---|---|---|---|---|---|
| Kim et al,[25] 2013, RCT | 137 ambulatory women aged ≥75 y with knee pain | Four groups. Exercise: twice-weekly group exercise for strength and balance. Exercise+: exercise and heat treatments. Heat only. Health education only | VAS, TUG, gait speed, Japanese Knee OA Measure | Facility based; 3 mo | Exercise+ showed greater improvement in pain intensity; gait speed and TUG improved in both exercise groups, although increase in TUG did not surpass the MDC |
| Levy et al,[26] 2012, single-group repeated measures | Adults aged ≥18 y with joint pain. Results shown for subgroup (n = 79) of older adults | Fitness and Exercise for People with Arthritis: group program incorporating strength, flexibility, agility, and aerobic conditioning exercises | TUG, 6MWT, AIMS 2, NRS, ASES | Facility based; 3 mo | Significant improvement in TUG, 6MWT, and pain intensity; no change in AIMS 2 physical function or affect scores; change in TUG and 6MWT did not exceed MDC |
| Maiers et al,[28] 2012, RCT | 241 community-dwelling adults aged ≥65 y with mechanical neck pain | Home exercise: 4 educational sessions on pain management with individualized exercise prescription with progression, followed by home exercise; exercises included flexibility, balance, coordination, trunk strength, and endurance. SMT + home exercise: exercise as above plus up to 20 chiropractor-delivered SMT sessions Supervised exercise: home exercise plus 20 1-h supervised exercise sessions | NRS, Neck Disability Index, SF 36, global improvement in pain, TUG | Home and facility based; 12 wk with 26-wk and 52-wk follow-up | All groups showed some improvement in Neck Disability Index with no between-group differences; SMT showed better improvement in pain than home exercise or supervised exercise; SMT was superior to home exercise in global improvement ratings; no changes in SF-36 or TUG scores; improvements in pain ratings from baseline were not sustained at 52 wk |

(continued on next page)

**Table 3**
*(continued)*

| Study | Participants | Interventions | Outcome Measures | Setting and Duration | Major Results |
|---|---|---|---|---|---|
| Messier et al,[29] 2004, RCT | 316 community-dwelling obese and overweight adults aged ≥60 y with knee pain and diagnosis of knee OA | Exercise only: walking at 50%–75% of HRR + resistance training Diet: 16 dietary weight loss sessions, including group and individual sessions Diet + exercise: exercise and diet interventions Healthy lifestyle control: 3 monthly meetings for education sessions then phone contacts | WOMAC, 6MWT, timed stair climb | Facility based for 4 mo, combined facility and home based for 2 more months, then 12 mo of home based | Diet + exercise group showed improved physical function scores on WOMAC and 6MWT; exercise only and diet only did not improve more than healthy lifestyle control; pain scale of WOMAC improved the most for diet + exercise group |
| Parker et al,[24] 2011, single-group repeated measures | 112 adults with noncancer pain aged ≥60 y stratified by race/ethnicity: African American, Hispanic, Non-Hispanic white | Arthritis Foundation's Self-help Program: Spanish language version incorporated exercise, including stretching, endurance, and relaxation | NRS, PSEQ exercise uptake | Senior center based; 6 wk | Significant reduction in pain intensity but not more than the MDC; all groups showed increased exercise at 3-mo follow-up with largest exercise uptake by Hispanic subjects who also showed greatest improvement in pain self-efficacy |
| Simmons et al,[49] 2002, RCT | 51 incontinent residents of a skilled nursing facility aged ≥65 y | Intervention group: walking or wheelchair mobility plus 8 repetitions of sit-to-stand Control group: no exercise | 30-s chair rise; distance walked/wheeled in 10 min, modified Geriatric Pain Measures, count of verbal and nonverbal pain behaviors during endurance tasks | Facility based; 32 wk | No change in pain reports; improved 30-s chair rise compared with control |

| Study | Subjects | Intervention | Measures | Setting | Results |
|---|---|---|---|---|---|
| Tse et al,[50] 2011, single-group repeated measures | 75 nursing home residents, 55 with chronic pain | Group-based exercise: intervention included strengthening, stretching, balance, and coordination exercises with encouragement to exercise independently between sessions | Cantonese Verbal Rating Scale for pain intensity, Barthel ADL Index, Elderly Mobility Scale | Facility based; 8 wk | Subjects with pain at baseline had a 2-point reduction in pain intensity, significantly improved mobility, but no change in ADL |
| Weiner et al,[51] 2008, RCT | 200 adults with chronic low back pain aged ≥65 y | PENS: 30 min of electrical stimulation through 10 needles PENS+: PENS treatment plus a general conditioning and aerobic exercise class with home exercise Control PENS: subthreshold PENS treatment Control PENS + exercise | McGill Pain Questionnaire; Pain thermometer; RMDQ; Physical Activity Scale for the Elderly; gait speed; 5× chair rise; timed stair climb; PSEQ; FABQ | Facility based with home component; 6 wk | All groups showed a significant decrease in pain intensity, improvement in gait speed, reduction in disability; exercise did not enhance pain reduction or functional improvement beyond that achieved with PENS and control PENS; subjects in the exercise groups achieved significant reduction in fear avoidance beliefs sustained at a 6-mo follow-up |

*Abbreviations:* ADL, activities of Daily Living; AIMS 2; Arthritis Impact Measurement Scales 2; ASES, Arthritis Self-efficacy Scale; FABQ, Fear Avoidance Beliefs Questionnaire; Geri-AIMS, Geriatric AIMS; PENS, percutaneous electrical nerve stimulation; PSEQ, Pain Self-efficacy Questionnaire; SMT, Spinal Manipulative Therapy.
*Data from* Refs.[22–26,28,29,48–51]

adherence were not noted. Further research on the impact of session frequency and intensity on pain-related outcomes will help develop optimal programming.

## PSYCHOLOGICAL INTERVENTION AND EXERCISE

Three trials contained a significant psychological intervention in addition to an exercise program (**Table 4**). Cognitive behavioral approaches were incorporated into 2 trials,[30,31] and motivational interviewing was applied in the third.[27] The efficacy of both types of psychological interventions in pain management has been established.[32–35] Thus, these techniques may offer an additional level of pain management beyond exercise alone. Therefore, it is important to assess the effects of these interventions combined with exercise in a separate portion of this article.

Cognitive behavior therapy is based in cognitive-social learning theory and can be used to increase patients' control over their own symptoms.[33] Self-efficacy is enhanced through a variety of psychological techniques that are psychoeducational in nature, and encourage patients to adopt a self-management approach to controlling their pain.[33] Motivational interviewing is a patient-centered technique that also seeks to encourage patient self-management of a problem through commitment to behavioral changes.[35]

Although none of these studies were specific with regard to the progression of exercise, nor did they seem to be based on established guidelines, taken together, they show the potential efficacy of a combined approach for chronic pain management. Of note, in addition to improvements in pain measures, all 3 studies reported significant improvements in pain self-efficacy. Self-management of pain is the goal of both motivational interviewing and cognitive behavior therapy, so improvement in self-efficacy is an important indicator of program success.

## AQUATICS

The buoyancy of the aquatic environment lessens impact on the joints and therefore seems an optimal exercise environment for individuals who have pain. Surprisingly, there were only 4 studies investigating the effect of aquatic exercise on pain in older adults with pain problems (**Table 5**).[36–39] It is interesting that some studies specifically targeting older adults with chronic pain emphasized fall risk and physical function. One study is included in our review because pain-related measures were included as outcome variables,[38] whereas the other collected these data but did not report post-intervention changes.[36]

The studies using aquatic exercise all enrolled older adults with lower extremity (LE) OA. The exercise programs were all modeled after programs delivered by community organizations, provided in a group format 2 times per week, but with varied length and intensity. Most incorporated the use of equipment (eg, floats and paddles) to increase resistance. Each program incorporated warm-up, motions to increase strength, balance-oriented activities, stepping/walking movements, and a cool-down. Other components varied by program.

Although positive outcomes were reported in 2 of the studies, our analysis showed that only 1 study[39] reported changes that surpassed the MDC for 1 pain-related outcome measure (the chair rise test). Other studies used the Western Ontario and McMaster Universities Arthritis Index (WOMAC) measures that did not exceed MDCs, or tests for which no standards were identified. Therefore, although the use of aquatic exercise for individuals with pain conditions is theoretically appealing, there is currently little evidence to support its use in geriatric pain management. However, because community-based aquatic exercise programs are widely available, they

**Table 4**
Combined exercise and psychological intervention studies

| Study | Participants | Interventions | Outcome Measures | Setting and Duration | Major Results |
|---|---|---|---|---|---|
| Beissner et al,[31] 2012, single-group repeated measures | 69 older adults aged ≥60 y with chronic back pain | Intervention group: Moving Past Pain program included both CBT and exercise components, including stretching, strengthening, and walking techniques | RMDQ, NRS, PSEQ, ADL score | 8 wk of group intervention at a facility | Combined groups and Hispanic group had reduced RMDQ more than the MDC; Hispanic group had reduced pain more than the MDC and the combined group had significant decrease; combined groups and Hispanic group had improvement in pain self-efficacy (PSEQ) |
| Nicholas et al,[30] 2013, RCT | 141 adults with chronic pain aged ≥65 y | CBT plus exercise: group sessions with psychologist using cognitive behavioral approach followed by stretching, aerobic, functional, and strengthening exercises with home exercise encouraged. Exercise Attention Control: Exercises as more than but no encouragement for home exercise and cognitive behavioral intervention; Wait list control | Modified RMDQ, NRS, pain-related distress measured on 11-point scale, 6MWT, functional reach | Facility based; 4 wk | CBT plus exercise fared better in terms of pain disability, pain-related distress, functional reach; more subjects in the CBT plus exercise group achieved meaningful change in disability than in the control groups |
| Tse et al,[27] 2013, RCT | 56 adults aged ≥65 y with chronic musculoskeletal pain | Intervention group: motivational interviewing and exercise, including stretching and strengthening; an HEP was provided. Control group: participation in usual center programs | NRS, PSEQ, EMS | 8 wk of group intervention at a facility, with a provided HEP | Significant reductions in NRS for the intervention group; significant improvements in self-efficacy (PSEQ) and EMS scores for the intervention group |

*Abbreviation:* CBT, cognitive behavior therapy.
Data from Refs.[27,30,31]

**Table 5**
**Aquatic exercise**

| Study | Participants | Interventions | Outcome Measures | Setting and Duration | Major Results |
|-------|--------------|---------------|------------------|----------------------|---------------|
| Arnold et al,[36] 2011, RCT | 54 adults aged ≥65 y with hip pain, diagnosed hip OA, and ≥1 fall risk factors | Exercise only: aquatic exercise for stretching, strengthening, trunk control, posture, and balance. Exercise+ group also received education for balance self-efficacy and transition to land-based exercise | 6MWT, Physical Activity Scale for the Elderly; AIMS 2 | Facility based; 11 wk | No pain outcomes were reported; some improvement in falls self-efficacy |
| Cochrane et al,[37] 2005, RCT | 312 adults aged ≥60 y with confirmed LE OA | Intervention: group-based water exercises designed for similarity to programs offered in community. Planned progressions were included Control: usual care and a quarterly telephone interview | WOMAC; SF-36; EuroQol VAS; gait speed and timed stair climb | Facility based; 12 mo | Intervention group showed significant improvements in pain and self-reported functioning at 12 mo, but effects were not significant at 6 mo after program completion; gait speed and stair climb times were improved in the exercise groups; only 53% complied with the program |

| Study | Population | Intervention | Outcome measures | Setting; duration | Results |
|---|---|---|---|---|---|
| Hale et al,[38] 2012, RCT | 35 ambulatory adults aged ≥65 y with self-reported LE OA and 1 or more fall risk factors | Intervention: self-paced aquatic exercise with balance component; Control: 1-h computer skills training | TUG, WOMAC; AIMS 2 | Facility based; 12 wk | No change in any pain-related outcome measure |
| Lau et al,[39] 2014, single-group repeated measures | 20 community-dwelling adults aged ≥65 y with physician-diagnosed knee OA | Education + aquatic exercise for strength, range of motion, balance | CAIMS 2; 6MWT; 30-s chair rise | Facility based; 10 wk | Improved mobility, pain intensity, mood, and level of tension (from CAIMS 2); improved 30-s chair rise; improvement in 6MWT did not exceed the MDC |

*Abbreviation:* CAIMS 2, Chinese AIMS 2.
*Data from* Refs.[36-39]

constitute a viable option for older adults who wish to sustain or increase their level of physical activity in a low-impact environment.

## OTHER EXERCISE MODALITIES

The other category includes movement-based interventions that do not fit in any of the groups discussed earlier. Two studies on tai chi[40,41] and one on agility exercises[14] are reviewed here (**Table 6**).

Tai chi is a form of exercise with roots in Chinese martial arts. The practice of tai chi entails moving through a series of slow, gentle, continuous movements and has commonly been studied for its effects on balance and general health in older adults. Tai chi has been shown to be a safe exercise method in older adults and contains elements of balance training, strengthening, concentration, and postural alignment, allowing it to target multiple body systems.[42,43] Despite the safe, multimodal training it provides, tai chi has not been studied extensively as a method of pain management in older adults. Of the 186 results returned in a PubMed search containing the terms "Tai Chi" and "older adults," only 2 addressed pain and met our inclusion criteria.[40,41] The rationale for agility training as an intervention for individuals with pain is less clear, but this type of exercise is available in the community and therefore presents an option for group exercise.

All 3 studies reported positive outcomes in terms of pain and disability, but these results must be interpreted with caution. Our analysis revealed that no outcome achieved a mean improvement beyond established MDCs or MCIDs. Furthermore, the ability to generalize from the tai chi results is limited, because one study enrolled a targeted population (ie, older adults with cognitive impairment and knee OA),[40] and the other included a sample of older adults who were not complaining of pain at the time of enrollment.[41]

## SUMMARY

From this review of movement-based therapies it seems that exercise has its strongest impact on function, with improvements in both self-report and performance measures of function being found regardless of exercise type. Although some studies report a decrease in pain intensity following an exercise-based or movement-based treatment, this evidence is less consistent. Importantly, there is no evidence of increased pain with exercise, which is important because fear of pain presents as a barrier to uptake of movement-based therapies.

Adherence is an important consideration for any exercise program, because benefits dissipate when exercise is not sustained. In a study of the long-term outcomes of individualized progressive exercise performed twice weekly by community-dwelling older adults with chronic back pain, Mailloux and colleagues[44] found that participants who adhered to home exercises had improved disability scores 2 years after discharge compared with those who discontinued exercise. This finding is consistent with those from group exercise programs,[22,23,45] reinforcing the importance of addressing patient barriers to adopting exercise as a long-term pain management strategy. Common barriers include lack of time, fear of exacerbating pain, lack of perceived need, and simple lack of motivation. Many of these barriers can be successfully addressed with careful listening, troubleshooting, and patient education. **Box 5** includes some motivation tips that can be shared with patients. Asking patients about their exercise habits at each visit also helps to hold them accountable.

There are several limitations to the literature on movement-based therapies for older adults with pain. First, for the exercise interventions for which published parameter

**Table 6**
Other exercise modalities

| Study | Participants | Interventions | Outcome Measures | Setting and Duration | Major Results |
|---|---|---|---|---|---|
| Liu-Ambrose et al,[14] 2005, RCT | 98 nonexercising white women aged 75–85 y with diagnosis of osteoporosis or osteopenia | Resistance group: free-weight training for UEs, LEs, and trunk at 50%–60% 1RM progressing to 75%–85% 1RM<br>Agility group: dance moves, obstacle courses, ball games<br>Control group: stretching and relaxation exercises | ODQ, QUALEFFO | Facility-based group exercise for 25 wk | All 3 groups improved on the ODQ with no between-group differences; resistance and agility groups showed improved QUALEFFO score with no between-group differences; compliance was 85% in the resistance group |
| Ross et al,[41] 1999, single-group repeated measures | 17 adults aged 69–92 y | Intervention group: 18 classes of tai chi provided by a trained instructor 3× weekly | VAS pain with AROM, sit-and-reach test, tandem walk, single-leg balance time | Group exercise provided at a facility for 6 wk | VAS-measured pain with AROM was reduced significantly; nonsignificant improvements were seen in flexibility, balance, and postural sway |
| Tsai et al,[40] 2013, cluster randomized trial | 55 adults aged ≥60 y with subtle to moderate cognitive impairment and knee OA | Intervention group: 12-form Sun Tai Chi for arthritis 3× weekly, provided by trained instructor<br>Control group: health education, culture-related activities, and other social activities | WOMAC, modified TUG, 5× sit-to-stand test | Group exercise at a facility for 20 wk | Statistically significant difference in WOMAC pain scores was seen from week 9 on, favoring tai chi group, but study was underpowered for all physical performance measures |

*Abbreviation:* AROM, active range of motion.
*Data from* Refs.[14,40,41]

---

**Box 5**
**Motivation tips**

- Exercise with a friend, and hold each other accountable
- Use a calendar to log your exercise
- Set goals for exercise and reward yourself when goals are met
- Use a smartphone fitness app that provides prompts for exercise
- Switch up your routine to prevent boredom; for example, change the walking route or try an exercise class
- Pick exercises that you enjoy, so you have fun while working out

---

guidelines exist, most of the studies did not adhere to the guidelines. Dosing of exercise intensity was consistently less than recommended, likely leading to a subtherapeutic training stimulus. Physical stress theory asserts that sufficient stress (intensity) must be imparted on a tissue or system to incur positive adaptation.[17] The lack of sufficient intensity may have contributed to the lack of clinically meaningful change in pain outcome measures seen across most of the resistance and aerobic training studies. It is likely that understimulation of older adults during exercise is caused by fears that older adults cannot or will not tolerate greater intensity of exercise. This fear perhaps reflects ageist or paternalistic attitudes, which paradoxically diminish the potential for optimal function. However, an AGS consensus document asserts that intensities of up to 80% of 1RM for resistance training and 60% of maximum heart rate/maximum oxygen uptake are safe for older adults with OA related pain.[2] The caveat is that older adults must be appropriately screened for any contraindications and the exercise must be progressed appropriately to the high intensity level to ensure patient safety. In this article, it was not possible to draw conclusions regarding the dose-response relationship between exercise and pain, because no study compared varying levels of exercise intensity. This deficit in the literature was also identified in a 2006 review.[3]

Appropriate progression of exercise is another important component of exercise training.[2] The lack of clear progression schema was a recurrent theme in the studies reviewed. Progression ensures that the patient's physiologic systems remain appropriately stressed, allowing positive adaptation to continue. An AGS consensus document regarding exercise for pain management in older adults with knee OA suggests that, following an acclimation period to exercise, isometric exercises should be progressed gradually from 30% to 75% of muscle maximum voluntary contraction, isometric resistance training is appropriately progressed by increasing resistance by 5% to 10% weekly, and aerobic intensity or volume can be increased by 2.5% per week.[2]

Another limitation of the literature was the paucity of studies incorporating pain-related outcome measures for some of the commonly recommended exercise types, including aquatics, tai chi, and yoga. Studies using these formats often included younger adults, so it was impossible to determine the separate impact on older adults. Further research examining the impact of these forms of exercise on older adults with pain problems will be helpful in making appropriate exercise recommendations.

Despite these limitations, it is clear that appropriately dosed exercise is beneficial to older adults with pain, so health care providers should recommend regular exercise for all patients with pain.[2] Exercise guidelines include strength training, aerobic conditioning, and flexibility exercises for optimal results. Given the importance of adherence and the variable exercise preferences, barriers, and facilitators among older adults, flexibility in prescribing exercise is critical to success, because performance is affected by multiple health and related factors.[46,47]

When feasible, prescriptions for movement-based therapies should incorporate individualized measures of intensity and also specify appropriate frequency and duration of exercise bouts. Sedentary individuals can begin with small bouts of exercise (eg, 10 minutes) and gradually increase time and intensity. Patients with little exercise experience, or those with fears related to movement, may benefit from guidance on correct exercise technique, either through work with a physical therapist or a personal trainer who has experience working with this population. Group class instructors can also provide guidance on correct form. Classes can often be found through local YMCAs, senior centers, and community centers. Some gyms provide land-based and/or water-based exercise classes specifically designed for older adults, with instructors who are attuned to the needs of this population. Individuals with no access to fitness facilities can engage in home exercise with little or no equipment. The Arthritis Foundation Web site is an excellent source for exercise tips and sample routines. Although not specific to pain, the American Diabetes Association Web site provides exercise education, and the Centers for Disease Control and Prevention has a well-developed strength training section, as well as education on other forms of exercise.

## REFERENCES

1. Johnson M, Martinson M. Efficacy of electrical nerve stimulation for chronic musculoskeletal pain: a meta-analysis of randomized controlled trials. Pain 2007;130(1–2):157–65.
2. American Geriatrics Society Panel on Exercise and Osteoarthritis. Exercise prescription for older adults with osteoarthritis pain: consensus practice recommendations. J Am Geriatr Soc 2001;49(6):808–23.
3. Focht BC. Effectiveness of exercise interventions in reducing pain symptoms among older adults with knee osteoarthritis: a review. J Aging Phys Act 2006; 14(2):212–35.
4. Gloth MJ, Matesi AM. Physical therapy and exercise in pain management. Clin Geriatr Med 2001;17(3):525–35.
5. Roddy E, Zhang W, Doherty M, et al. Evidence-based recommendations for the role of exercise in the management of osteoarthritis of the hip or knee—the MOVE consensus. Rheumatology (Oxford) 2005;44(1):67–73.
6. Pescatello LS, American College of Sports Medicine. ACSM's guidelines for exercise testing and prescription. Philadelphia: Wolters Kluwer; Lippincott Williams; Wilkins Health; 2014.
7. Nijs J, Thielemans A. Kinesiophobia and symptomatology in chronic fatigue syndrome: a psychometric study of two questionnaires. Psychol Psychother 2008; 81(3):273–83.
8. Fuentes CJ, Armijo-Olivo S, Magee DJ, et al. Effects of exercise therapy on endogenous pain-relieving peptides in musculoskeletal pain: a systematic review. Clin J Pain 2011;27(4):365–74.
9. Beckwée D, Vaes P, Cnudde M, et al. Osteoarthritis of the knee: why does exercise work? a qualitative study of the literature. Ageing Res Rev 2013;12(1): 226–36.
10. Petrella RJ, Bartha C. Home based exercise therapy for older patients with knee osteoarthritis: a randomized clinical trial. J Rheumatol 2000;27(9):2215–21.

11. Hasegawa M, Yamazaki S, Kimura M, et al. Community-based exercise program reduces chronic knee pain in elderly Japanese women at high risk of requiring long-term care: a non-randomized controlled trial. Geriatr Gerontol Int 2013; 13(1):167–74.

12. Wong YK, Hui E, Woo J. A community-based exercise programme for older persons with knee pain using telemedicine. J Telemed Telecare 2005;11(6):310–5.

13. Ettinger WH Jr, Burns R, Messier SP, et al. A randomized trial comparing aerobic exercise and resistance exercise with a health education program in older adults with knee osteoarthritis: the fitness arthritis and seniors trial (fast). JAMA 1997; 277(1):25–31.

14. Liu-Ambrose TY, Khan KM, Eng JJ, et al. Both resistance and agility training reduce back pain and improve health-related quality of life in older women with low bone mass. Osteoporos Int 2005;16(11):1321–9.

15. Murphy SL, Strasburg DM, Lyden AK, et al. Effects of activity strategy training on pain and physical activity in older adults with knee or hip osteoarthritis: a pilot study. Arthritis Care Res 2008;59(10):1480–7.

16. Lim CG, Lee S, Ko E, et al. Effect of a complex exercise program for the lower extremities on quadriceps activity and pain of elderly patients with knee osteoarthritis: a pilot study. J Phys Ther Sci 2013;25(3):249–51.

17. Mueller MJ, Maluf KS. Tissue adaptation to physical stress: a proposed "Physical stress theory" to guide physical therapist practice, education, and research. Phys Ther 2002;82(4):383–403.

18. Nyrop KA, Muss HB, Hackney B, et al. Feasibility and promise of a 6-week program to encourage physical activity and reduce joint symptoms among elderly breast cancer survivors on aromatase inhibitor therapy. J Geriatr Oncol 2014; 5(2):148–55.

19. Talbot LA, Gaines JM, Huynh TN, et al. A home-based pedometer-driven walking program to increase physical activity in older adults with osteoarthritis of the knee: a preliminary study. J Am Geriatr Soc 2003;51(3):387–92.

20. Rhudy JL, Dubbert PM, Kirchner KA, et al. Efficacy of a program to encourage walking in VA elderly primary care patients: the role of pain. Psychol Health Med 2007;12(3):289–98.

21. Ferrell BA, Josephson KR, Pollan AM, et al. A randomized trial of walking versus physical methods for chronic pain management. Aging (Milano) 1997;9(1–2): 99–105.

22. Hughes SL, Seymour RB, Campbell RT, et al. Long-term impact of Fit and Strong! on older adults with osteoarthritis. Gerontologist 2006;46(6):801–14.

23. Hughes SL, Seymour RB, Campbell R, et al. Impact of the Fit and Strong intervention on older adults with osteoarthritis. Gerontologist 2004;44(2):217–28.

24. Parker SJ, Vasquez R, Chen EK, et al. A comparison of the arthritis foundation self-help program across three race/ethnicity groups. Ethn Dis 2011;21(4): 444–50.

25. Kim H, Suzuki T, Saito K, et al. Effectiveness of exercise with or without thermal therapy for community-dwelling elderly Japanese women with non-specific knee pain: a randomized controlled trial. Arch Gerontol Geriatr 2013;57(3):352–9.

26. Levy SS, Macera CA, Hootman JM, et al. Evaluation of a multi-component group exercise program for adults with arthritis: fitness and exercise for people with arthritis (FEPA). Disabil Health J 2012;5(4):305–11.

27. Tse MM, Vong SK, Tang SK. Motivational interviewing and exercise programme for community-dwelling older persons with chronic pain: a randomised controlled study. J Clin Nurs 2013;22(13–14):1843–56.

28. Maiers M, Bronfort G, Evans R, et al. OA06.03. Spinal manipulative therapy, supervised rehabilitative exercise and home exercise for seniors with neck pain. BMC Complement Altern Med 2012;12:1.

29. Messier SP, Loeser RF, Miller GD, et al. Exercise and dietary weight loss in overweight and obese older adults with knee osteoarthritis: the arthritis, diet, and activity promotion trial. Arthritis Rheum 2004;50(5):1501–10.

30. Nicholas MK, Asghari A, Blyth FM, et al. Self-management intervention for chronic pain in older adults: a randomised controlled trial. Pain 2013;154(6):824–35.

31. Beissner K, Parker SJ, Henderson CR Jr, et al. A cognitive-behavioral plus exercise intervention for older adults with chronic back pain: race/ethnicity effect? J Aging Phys Act 2012;20(2):246–65.

32. Morley S, Eccleston C, Williams A. Systematic review and meta-analysis of randomized controlled trials of cognitive behaviour therapy and behaviour therapy for chronic pain in adults, excluding headache. Pain 1999;80(1–2):1–13.

33. Kerns RD, Otis JD, Marcus KS. Cognitive-behavioral therapy for chronic pain in the elderly. Clin Geriatr Med 2001;17(3):503–23.

34. Jensen MP, Nielson WR, Kerns RD. Toward the development of a motivational model of pain self-management. J Pain 2003;4(9):477–92.

35. Vong SK, Cheing GL, Chan F, et al. Motivational enhancement therapy in addition to physical therapy improves motivational factors and treatment outcomes in people with low back pain: a randomized controlled trial. Arch Phys Med Rehabil 2011;92(2):176–83.

36. Arnold CM, Faulkner RA, Gyurcsik NC. The relationship between falls efficacy and improvement in fall risk factors following an exercise plus educational intervention for older adults with hip osteoarthritis. Physiother Can 2011;63(4):41–420.

37. Cochrane T, Davey RC, Matthes Edwards SM. Randomised controlled trial of the cost-effectiveness of water-based therapy for lower limb osteoarthritis. Health Technol Assess 2005;9(31):iii–iv, ix–xi, 1–114.

38. Hale LA, Waters D, Herbison P. A randomized controlled trial to investigate the effects of water-based exercise to improve falls risk and physical function in older adults with lower-extremity osteoarthritis. Arch Phys Med Rehabil 2012;93(1): 27–34.

39. Lau MC, Lam JK, Siu E, et al. Physiotherapist-designed aquatic exercise programme for community-dwelling elders with osteoarthritis of the knee: a Hong Kong pilot study. Hong Kong Med J 2014;20(1):16–23.

40. Tsai PF, Chang JY, Beck C, et al. A pilot cluster-randomized trial of a 20-week tai chi program in elders with cognitive impairment and osteoarthritic knee: effects on pain and other health outcomes. J Pain Symptom Manage 2013;45(4):660–9.

41. Ross MC, Bohannon AS, Davis DC, et al. The effects of a short-term exercise program on movement, pain, and mood in the elderly. Results of a pilot study. J Holist Nurs 1999;17(2):139–47.

42. Wu G. Evaluation of the effectiveness of tai chi for improving balance and preventing falls in the older population—A review. J Am Geriatr Soc 2002;50(4): 746–54.

43. Wang C, Collet J, Lau J. The effect of tai chi on health outcomes in patients with chronic conditions: a systematic review. Arch Intern Med 2004;164(5):493–501.

44. Mailloux J, Finno M, Rainville J. Long-term exercise adherence in the elderly with chronic low back pain. Am J Phys Med Rehabil 2006;85(2):120–6.

45. van Gool CH, Penninx BW, Kempen GI, et al. Effects of exercise adherence on physical function among overweight older adults with knee osteoarthritis. Arthritis Rheum 2005;53(1):24–32.

46. Petursdottir U, Arnadottir SA, Halldorsdottir S. Facilitators and barriers to exercising among people with osteoarthritis: a phenomenological study. Phys Ther 2010;90(7):1014–25.

47. Rejeski WJ, Ettinger WH Jr, Martin K, et al. Treating disability in knee osteoarthritis with exercise therapy: a central role for self-efficacy and pain. Arthritis Care Res 1998;11(2):94–101.

48. Hasegawa R, Islam MM, Nasu E, et al. Effects of combined balance and resistance exercise on reducing knee pain in community-dwelling older adults. Phys Occup Ther Geriatr 2010;28(1):44–56.

49. Simmons SF, Ferrell BA, Schnelle JF. Effects of a controlled exercise trial on pain in nursing home residents. Clin J Pain 2002;18(6):380–5.

50. Tse MM, Wan VT, Ho SS. Physical exercise: does it help in relieving pain and increasing mobility among older adults with chronic pain? J Clin Nurs 2011; 20(5–6):635–44.

51. Weiner DK, Perera S, Rudy TE, et al. Efficacy of percutaneous electrical nerve stimulation and therapeutic exercise for older adults with chronic low back pain: a randomized controlled trial. Pain 2008;140(2):344–57.

# Psychological Approaches to Coping with Pain in Later Life

Christopher Eccleston, PhD*, Abby Tabor, PhD,
Rhiannon Terri Edwards, MSc, Edmund Keogh, PhD

## KEYWORDS

- Psychology • Cognitive behavioral therapy • Evidence • Older adults • Coping

## KEY POINTS

- Normal aging involves a balance between assimilative and accommodative coping. Knowing when to adjust and when to endure is crucial to healthy aging.
- Psychological therapies are promising in general, but only a few trials have been reported with older people, which show limited effect.
- Psychological therapies for chronic pain in older age will need to be based on a theory of fractured aging, and include innovations in cognitive therapy.

## INTRODUCTION

Dramatic changes to life expectancy have occurred in the last century, a progression accompanied by a changing pattern of disease and morbidity.[1] Understanding a normal process of aging and the experience of pain in this older patient group, for whom multimorbidity is the norm rather than the exception, presents a critical challenge to psychological approaches in health care.

Pain is a common feature of later life,[2] and people expect to hurt more as they age.[3] What is more surprising, however, is that it is not inevitable that pain will lead to suffering. There is enormous variety in how people attempt to adjust to the challenge of pain, what strategies inoculate against further pain and suffering, and how far one can intervene in successfully improving adjustment. For example, the prevalence of back pain does not increase with age, but the prevalence of disabling back pain does.[4] Additionally, those at greater risk of disability are more likely to have experienced primary depression[5,6] and loneliness.[6] Similar associations have been reported in other primary pain disorders such as fibromyalgia.[7] How one adapts to the challenge of pain is crucial to whether suffering dominates later life.

Disclosure Statement: The authors have nothing to disclose.
Centre for Pain Research, The University of Bath, Bath BA2 7AY, UK
* Corresponding author.
E-mail address: c.eccleston@bath.ac.uk

Clin Geriatr Med 32 (2016) 763–771
http://dx.doi.org/10.1016/j.cger.2016.06.004     geriatric.theclinics.com

This article presents an overview of normal aging from a psychological perspective, ending with a consideration of how one attempts to age optimally by promoting growth and reducing suffering. Using this model as a framework for treatment, the authors review the evidence for the efficacy and safety of psychological interventions for the management of chronic pain. Finally, the article summarizes the implications for future research and practice, and suggests areas for profitable development.

## NORMAL AGING AND ADJUSTMENT

The most successful model of normal human aging in later life, known as the dual-process model, focuses on motivation to protect, change, or achieve, valued goals.[8,9] It is a model of need, of striving, of motivation, and one that uses a language of goal pursuit and of the self-regulation of behavior.

At the heart of this motivational view of human development is the idea that one is always moving toward or away from desired goals. Although the goals may vary depending on one's phase of life, people are always gaining or losing. People attempt to put resources into ensuring that their goals are reached, or are alternatively working to mitigate the impact of their losses. From a coping perspective, one can classify all attempts at managing the discrepancy between what is striven for and what is achievable in 2 broad categories known as assimilative and accommodative modes.

Assimilative coping is when all efforts are made to alter the world to fit the goal, to alter one's own behavior and the behavior of others, and to change structural influences. It is all about making it happen. Accommodative coping is when the importance of an unachievable goal is reduced and replaced with an achievable one. When faced with any goal one has a simple choice: work hard to achieve it, or work hard to make the consequences of not achieving it less damaging. Imagine, for example, a concert pianist assimilating to pain on playing by learning to perform standing, altering hand positions, avoiding Chopin. But ultimately, accommodating to the loss of function by changing from a goal of playing to a goal of listening, critiquing, or teaching. These broadly defined dual processes, and how easily one can employ them, are not personality characteristics, and are not inherently fixed to particular problem presentations; they are context-dependent modes of problem solving. Central to this model of coping is the recognition that the needs, wants, and desires that define who we are change over time.

The challenge of coping is knowing when to assimilate and when to accommodate, whether to single-mindedly and tenaciously pursue a goal without concern for consequence (tenacious goal pursuit) or whether instead to flexibly disengage from any emotional investment in the goal (flexible goal adjustment). Typically people are able to use both modes of coping. For example, one investigation of how people react to negative life events in older age investigated the challenge of potentially competing modes of coping. Questionnaires were completed by 670 adults with a mean age of 74 years. People reported the negative stressful life events they had experienced, how they had attempted to cope, and their current affective state (depression). The results showed that older adults were able to use both modes effectively. However, less effort placed in these attempts to adjust—described as low tenacity and low flexibility—was associated with greater depression. Accommodative coping—being able to flexibly adjust away from the unachievable—appeared to protect against depression, especially when people had experienced multiple negative life events.[10]

Tenacious goal pursuit is a popular idea. It has been recently investigated in the study of achievement as grit, defined more subjectively as a desire and willingness to persevere in achieving a long-term goal.[11] Largely, what one thinks of as coping is assimilative coping: conscious attempts to change that involve effort to reach a goal.[12]

More complex is an understanding of accommodative coping, of how people disengage as they age. Accommodative coping is perhaps best thought of as a successful outcome rather than a strategy. What matters in accommodating is that in disengaging from a once-desired and fought-for goal, that this disengagement protects from affective distress, and does not fuel it: that the accommodation is not surrender, mental defeat, or depression. Older age, however, for many involves a shift away from concerns of personal achievement and future goals and a greater concern with core values that are beyond the individual, what has been called a final decentration.[13]

## FRACTURED AGING AND CHRONIC PAIN

The greater the number of physical health problems, the greater the subjective feeling of aging.[14] For those with multimorbidity and a high symptom burden, adjusting to a life dominated by aversive physical sensations is a significant challenge, a challenge that is often unmet. The approach to coping that the authors have called assimilative and accommodative has been described more engagingly in an in-depth qualitative study as the attempt to adjust and endure.[15] For many people, however, adjustment is not always possible, and endurance is a tremendous further burden. Both modes of coping can fail. The failure of coping attempts, however, are not global or random; they are often specific. And the more specific or stereotypical they are, the easier it is to design interventions that may help. There are 3 challenges to aging well with pain that the authors present as a threat to self (identity), a threat to mood (depression), and a threat to activity (disability).

### Identity

Identity is always at stake in chronic pain. Pain interrupts attention, interferes with current goals, and can challenge the identity of the person attempting to respond.[16] Although there has been much written about the first 2 aspects, there is surprisingly little research on the impact of chronic pain on identity. Chronic pain operates as an assault on the coherence of self, in particular of one's belief in mastery, competence, and performance. Patients also report that the effort spent in seeking legitimation for pain is a fatiguing further source of distress. Patients often experience the need to validate their experience and protect their identity as a person with control.[17] For some, a tenacious pursuit of this defense can lead to worry, perseverative coping (repeating the same failed strategy), and an inability to disengage from an unachievable goal. All energies go into finding a solution, often to an insoluble problem, a form of misdirected problem solving.[18,19] Over time, patients can become focused on a singular and narrow goal (eg, the return to a previous job role, seemingly oblivious to the fact that the role no longer exists to return to, or that even without pain the role would have expired naturally). The first challenge to aging well with pain is to counter the identity suspension, an altering of a natural course of subjective aging, that can occur as a result of perseverative misdirected problem solving, tenaciously pursued.

### Depression

Depression consistently emerges as a risk of living with pain in later life. There are data in community samples of patients with pain-related diseases such as osteoarthritis,[20] cancer,[21] and in samples where pain is part of a complex symptom profile associated with frailty.[22,23] Depression and the concomitant symptoms of depression such as anxiety, sleep disturbance, and social withdrawal are dominant concerns, especially among isolated older adults. There are some data showing that resilience to loss through accommodation, often measured as acceptance, may buffer against the effects of depression and pain.[24] However, acceptance of loss of agency, identity, and possible future goals has largely negative meanings for patients with pain. Acceptance is something to be suspicious of, because it is perceived as a form of social rejection or a sign of personal weakness; it is often experienced as pejorative.[25] Although academic psychology is interested in how acceptance is achieved, it is better thought of as an outcome rather than a strategy,[26] especially when one considers the general methods of measurement that assess a rather countercultural willingness to be in pain.[27] The second challenge of aging well with pain is to address the symptom burden of depression, not as a primary disorder, but in its relationship with pain. Too often, the disengagement of achievable goals is not acceptance, but depressive withdrawal.

### Disability

Disability, exacerbated by pain, depression, and sleep disturbance, is often the more visible outcome of a lack of successful adjustment to chronic pain. A major feature of disability in the older patient with chronic pain is a fear of falling and a pattern of avoidance behavior driven by that fear.[28] There is a relatively advanced understanding of avoidance behavior in the context of pain, but models have not yet incorporated falling and fear of falling.[29] Considered in the context of coping, it is unclear whether attempts at altering perceived risk factors for falling are adaptive or should be considered normal accommodative withdrawal. In addition, the perception of self-vulnerability and fragility that can emerge after a fall can exacerbate self-punishing cognition that is a classical feature of depression. To be clear, thoughts of worthlessness, unwanted dependency, loneliness, and reduced social stimulation provide a fertile ground for reduced function, fear of failure, and general social withdrawal and disability. The third challenge of aging well with pain is to recognize when disability develops as a consequence of avoidance versus physical frailty. People rarely act without purpose, so understanding what is blocking a goal is important. Often disability is the visible marker of a psychological struggle with a feared and uncertain future.

## PSYCHOLOGICAL INTERVENTIONS

Little is known about the people who adapt successfully to chronic pain, because they do not seek medical care for this issue. Many people are expert not only at assimilation, but also at assimilation within a broader context of personal growth.[30,31] Typically patients present with the 3 challenges to normal aging summarized previously as identity, depression, and disability. Psychological interventions are typically designed to alter these outcomes: to improve self-determined coping, to improve mood, and to increase engagement with valued activities. There are 3 main areas where psychological interventions have been developed that are relevant to coping with pain in older age. First there are studies specifically designed to increase the management of pain and its consequences. Second are the studies designed specifically to address depression including loneliness. And third, there is relevant literature on psychological interventions to reduce falling and fear of falling.

## COGNITIVE BEHAVIORAL THERAPY FOR CHRONIC PAIN

There is a long tradition of therapy development in the management of chronic pain and no shortage of randomized controlled trials and evaluations. The Cochrane review of randomized controlled trials (RCTs) for psychological interventions for adults reported small-to-medium effect sizes in outcome domains such as pain experience, depression, and disability.[32] The most recent update included a specific domain of worry and anxiety appraisal but found too little data to report. The meta-analyses reported were non-specific, focused on mean effects, and included trials of all adult treatments.

Only 3 trials were included that were specifically with older patients. One large trial recruited 218 older adults with an average age of 81.8 into a comparison between a simple education program and a multimodal pain management program.[33] In this study, there were no overall improvements in pain, disability, or depression. The authors speculate that this may be due to the inclusion of a mixed sample of different pain problems, and focusing on one specific area might help. Two other trials were included in the review that focused specifically on osteoarthritis, with mean ages of 64 and 63 years of age. In this specific treatment, the effects were more promising, showing small improvements,[34,35] although these improvements were not maintained at follow-up.[36,37] The idea of becoming more specific about the treatment and the population is sensible; the heterogeneity caused by combining individual studies can obscure specific effects. However, when one disaggregates these large studies, there are few data left. The authors recently undertook a systematic review of psychological treatments for adults with neuropathic pain. Given the rising age-related incidence of painful diabetic neuropathy (PDN) and postherpetic neuralgia (PHN), one would expect research attention. In fact, there are no RCTs of psychological treatments for PDN or PHN. The authors found only 2 studies, one in spinal cord injury and one in burning mouth syndrome. Worryingly, there is almost no evidence of the effectiveness and safety of psychological interventions for chronic neuropathic pain[38]; the field is best characterized as undeveloped.

Despite the gaps in the evidence base, some investigators see cause for optimism.[39] This optimism comes from an observation that treatments appear to be effective in general adult populations, and that older populations that find them credible stay engaged with the treatment trials. However, to date there is little guidance on the specific content or mode of delivery that might be useful. Early studies of mindfulness protocols are reported as positive,[40] however, the efficacy data lack promise. Other studies use fairly standard cognitive behavioral therapy (CBT) protocols. In terms of mode of delivery, 1 well conducted Australian trial showed that primary care delivery is possible, maybe even desirable.[41] A second study demonstrated that delivery by nonpsychologists is an important method to consider.[42] Possible e-health innovations are at an early stage of development. Until one can be more specific about content, their utility remains speculative.[43]

Psychological protocols that focus on specific aspects of the context of living or care, such as the risk of isolation and loneliness, are also promising. For example, working with peers may prove effective.[44,45] Similarly, a focus on activity engagement and falls prevention is likely to be a critical part of any psychological therapy that has engagement with valued goals and activities as an outcome. There is evidence for the reduction of risk of falling by altering structural barriers,[46] but also critically through understanding how fear of falling may be more disabling than falling itself.[47]

## NEXT-GENERATION COGNITIVE BEHAVIORAL THERAPY FOR THE TREATMENT OF CHRONIC PAIN IN OLDER ADULTS

The authors share the optimism that CBT, appropriately tailored, could be effective. What has been attempted to date has been less about the needs of the older person, and more an application of what is thought to work in general applied to an older

**Table 1**
**Adjust or endure: the challenges of pain to adaptive aging**

|  | Challenge | Therapy Content |
|---|---|---|
| Identity | Identify possible identity suspension/fracture: an altering of a natural course of subjective aging, characterized by perseverative misdirected problem solving, often tenaciously pursued despite failure | Cognitive therapy that focuses on experimenting with alternatives to closely held core beliefs, especially about acceptable old age; narrative content on the choices of values and actions |
| Depression | Identify symptom burden of depression, not as a primary disorder, but in its relationship with pain; too often, the disengagement of achievable goals is not acceptance, but depressive withdrawal | Content focused on reducing the influence of negative social emotions such as shame and embarrassment; techniques to promote self-compassion and self-forgiveness, in particular regard to self-determination biases |
| Disability | Identify when inactivity is avoidance, not physical frailty; assess what is blocking a goal Disability can be the visible marker of a psychological struggle with a feared and uncertain future | A focus on targets of avoidance beyond pain, such as falling and a focus on activity engagement and postural confidence; content aimed specifically at the risk of isolation and loneliness |

population: tailoring by sample but not by method or mode of delivery. And in some critical areas, such as chronic neuropathic pain, there is no evidence. What is needed is a better understanding of how to tailor psychological therapies to the challenges that chronic pain brings to normal aging. **Table 1** summarizes the possible areas of therapy development based on the idea that pain threatens identity, risks depression, and can effectively speed psychological aging by imposing disability. Although speculative, this model of interrupted normal aging suggests that treatment innovation can be improved with research on augmented cognitive therapy that focuses on experimenting with alternatives to closely held core beliefs, especially about acceptable old age.[48] Similarly, depression complicated by pain may need content focused on negative social emotions such as shame and embarrassment; advancements in techniques to promote self-compassion and self-forgiveness are promising.[49,50] Gaining an insight into the evolving expectations of normal aging and the associated experiences, both from the perspective of the patient and the health care professional, will form an important part of this exploration. Finally, advances in falls prevention research provide a positive approach to harm reduction in this patient population.

## SUMMARY

Psychological interventions for chronic pain in later life are promising in general, but have yet to show meaningful clinical benefit in older age. Novel psychological therapies should be guided by a model of pain as an alteration—a fracture—in normal aging. Targets of CBT need to broaden out of pain to multiple embodied sensations experienced within a context of a personal narrative of normal aging.[51]

## REFERENCES

1. Howse K. Increasing life expectancy and the compression of morbidity: a critical review of the debate: working paper no. 206. Oxford (United Kingdom): Oxford Institute of Ageing; University of Oxford; 2006.

2. Patel KV, Guralnik JM, Dansie EJ, et al. Prevalence and impact of pain among older adults in the United States: findings from the 2011 National Health and Aging Trends Study. Pain 2013;154:2649–57.
3. Sarkisian CA, Steers N, Hays RD, et al. Development of the 12-item expectations regarding aging survey. Gerontologist 2005;45:240–8.
4. Docking RE, Fleming J, Brayne C, et al. Epidemiology of back pain in older adults: prevalence and risk factors for back pain onset. Rheumatology 2011; 50:1645–53.
5. Reid MC, Williams CS, Concato J, et al. Depressive symptoms as a risk factor for disabling back pain in community-dwelling older person. J Am Geriatr Soc 2003; 51:1710–7.
6. Jacobs JM, Hsmmerman-Rozenberg R, Cohen A, et al. Chronic back pain among the elderly: prevalence, associations, and predictors. Spine 2006;31:e203–7.
7. McBeth J, Lacey RJ, Wilkie R. Predictors of new-onset widespread pain in older adults. Results from a population-based prospective cohort study in the UK. Arthritis Rheumatol 2014;66:757–67.
8. Brandtstädter J, Renner G. Tenacious goal pursuit and flexible goal adjustment: explication and age-related analysis of assimilative and accommodative strategies of coping. Psychol Aging 1990;5:58–67.
9. Brandtstädter J, Rothermund K. The life-course dynamics of goal pursuit and goal adjustment: a two process framework. Dev Rev 2002;22:117–50.
10. Bailly N, Joulain M, Hervé C, et al. Coping with negative life events in old age: the role of tenacious goal pursuit and flexible goal adjustment. Aging Ment Health 2012;16:431–7.
11. Duckworth A, Gross JJ. Self-control and grit: related but separable determinants of success. Curr Dir Psychol Sci 2014;23:319–25.
12. Skinner EA, Edge K, Altman J, et al. Searching for the structure of coping: a review and critique of category systems for classifying ways of coping. Psychol Bull 2003;129:216–69.
13. Brandtstädter J, Rothermund K, Kranz D, et al. Final decentrations: personal goals, rationality perspectives, and the awareness of life's finitude. Eur Psychol 2010;15:152–63.
14. Kotter-Grün D, Neupert SD, Stephan Y. Feeling old today? daily health, stressors, and affect explain day-to-day variability in subjective age. Psychol Health 2015; 30:1470–85.
15. Eckerblad J, Theander K, Ekdahl A, et al. To adjust and endure: a qualitative study of symptom burden in older people with multimorbidity. Appl Nurs Res 2015;28:322–7.
16. Eccleston C, Morley SJ, Williams AC. Psychological approaches to the chronic pain management: evidence and challenges. Br J Anaesth 2013;111:59–63.
17. Eccleston C, Williams AC, Rogers WS. Patients' and professionals' understandings of the causes of chronic pain: blame, responsibility, and identity protection. Soc Sci Med 1997;45:699–709.
18. Aldrich C, Eccleston C, Crombez G. Worrying about chronic pain: vigilance to threat and misdirected problem solving. Behav Res Ther 2000;38:457–70.
19. Eccleston C, Crombez G. Worry and chronic pain: a misdirected problem solving model. Pain 2007;132:233–6.
20. Hawker GA, Gignac MA, Badley E, et al. A longitudinal study to explain the pain-depression link in older adults with depression. Arthritis Care Res (Hoboken) 2011;10:1382–90.

21. Reyes-Gibby CC, Aday LA, Anderson KO, et al. Pain, depression, and fatigue in community-dwelling adults with and without a history of cancer. J Pain Symptom Manage 2006;32:118–28.

22. Blyth FM, Rochat S, Cumming RG, et al. Pain, frailty and comorbidity on older men: the CHAMP study. Pain 2008;140:224–30.

23. Shega JW, Dale W, Andrew M, et al. Persistent pain and frailty: a case for home-ostenosis. J Am Geriatr Soc 2011;60:113–7.

24. Shallcross AJ, Ford BQ, Floerke VA, et al. Getting better with age: the relationship between age, acceptance, and negative affect. J Pers Soc Psychol 2013;104:734–49.

25. Risdon A, Eccleston C, Crombez G, et al. How can we learn to live with pain? A Q-methodological analysis of the diverse understandings of acceptance of chronic pain. Soc Sci Med 2003;56:375–86.

26. Nicholas MK, Asghari A. Investigating acceptance in adjustment to chronic pain: is acceptance broader than we thought? Pain 2006;124:269–79.

27. Lauwerier E, Caes L, Van Damme S, et al. Acceptance questionnaires in patients with chronic pain: a content analysis. J Pain 2015;16:306–17.

28. Hadjistavropoulos T, Martin RR, Sharpe D, et al. A longitudinal investigation of fear of falling, fear of pain, and activity avoidance in community-dwelling older adults. J Aging Health 2007;19:965–84.

29. Crombez G, Eccleston C, Van Damme S, et al. Fear-avoidance model of chronic pain: the next generation. Clin J Pain 2012;28:475–83.

30. Phillips WJ, Ferguson SJ. Self-compassion: a resource for positive aging. J Gerontol B Psychol Sci Soc Sci 2013;68:529–39.

31. Pillemer K. 30 lessons for living: tried and true advice from the wisest Americans. New York: Penguin; 2013.

32. Williams AC, Eccleston C, Morley S. Psychological therapies for the management of chronic pain (excluding headache) in adults. Cochrane Database Syst Rev 2012;(11):CD007407.

33. Ersek M, Turner JA, Cain KC, et al. Results of a randomized controlled trial to examine the efficacy of a chronic pain self-management group for older adults [ISRCTN11899548]. Pain 2008;138:29–40.

34. Keefe FJ, Caldwell DS, Williams DA, et al. Pain coping skills training in the management of osteoarthritic knee pain: a comparative study. Behav Ther 1990;21:49–62.

35. Keefe FJ, Caldwell DS, Baucom D, et al. Spouse-assisted coping skills training in the management of osteoarthritic knee pain. Arthritis Care Res 1996;9:279–91.

36. Keefe FJ, Caldwell DS, Williams DA, et al. Pain coping skills training in the management of osteoarthritic knee pain: II. Follow-up results. Behav Ther 1990;21:435–47.

37. Keefe FJ, Caldwell DS, Baucom D, et al. Spouse-assisted coping skills training in the management of knee pain in osteoarthritis: long-term follow up results. Arthritis Care Res 1999;12:101–11.

38. Eccleston C, Hearn L, Williams AC. Psychological therapies for the management of chronic neuropathic pain in adults. Cochrane Database Syst Rev 2015;(10):CD011259.

39. McGuire BE, Nicholas MK, Asghari A, et al. The effectiveness of psychological treatments for chronic pain in older adults: cautious optimism and an agenda for research. Curr Opin Psychiatry 2014;27:380–4.

40. Morone ME, Greco CM, Moore CG, et al. A mind-body program for older adults with chronic low back pain: a randomized clinical trial. JAMA Internal Medicine 2016;176:329–37.
41. Nicholas MK, Asghari A, Blyth FM, et al. Self-management intervention for chronic pain in older adults: a randomized controlled trial. Pain 2013;154:824–35.
42. Broderick JE, Keefe FJ, Bruckenthal P, et al. Nurse practitioners can effectively deliver pain coping skills training to osteoarthritis patients with chronic pain: a randomized, controlled trial. Pain 2014;155:1743–54.
43. Eccleston C, Fisher E, Craig L, et al. Psychological therapies (Internet-delivered) for the management of chronic pain in adults. Cochrane Database Syst Rev 2014;(2):CD010152.
44. Tse MM, Vong SK, Ho SS. The effectiveness of an integrated pain management program for older persons and staff in nursing homes. Arch Gerontol Geriatr 2012;54:e203–12.
45. Tse MM, Lee PH, Ng SM, et al. Peer volunteers in an integrative pain management program for frail older adults with chronic pain: study protocol for a randomized controlled trial. Trials 2014;15:205.
46. Gillespie LD, Robertson MC, Gillespie WJ, et al. Interventions for preventing falls in older people living in the community. Cochrane Database Syst Rev 2012;(9):CD007146.
47. Delbaere K, Sturnieks DL, Crombez G, et al. Concern about falls elicits changes in gait parameters in conditions of postural threat in older people. J Gerontol A Biol Sci Med Sci 2009;64:237–42.
48. Beck AT, Dozois DJ. Cognitive therapy: current status and future directions. Annu Rev Med 2011;62:397–409.
49. Lumley MA, Sklar ER, Carty JN. Emotional disclosure interventions for chronic pain: from the laboratory to the clinic. Transl Behav Med 2012;2:73–81.
50. Leaviss J, Uttley L. Psychotherapeutic benefits of compassion-focused therapy: an early systematic review. Psychol Med 2015;45:927–45.
51. Eccleston C. Embodied: the psychology of physical sensation. Oxford (United Kingdom): Oxford University Press; 2016.

# Interventional Techniques for Management of Pain in Older Adults

Amber K. Brooks, MD[a],*, Mercy A. Udoji, MD, CMQ[b]

## KEYWORDS

- Interventional pain management • Chronic pain • Osteoarthritis • Steroid injection
- Osteoporosis • Vertebral compression fracture

## KEY POINTS

- Physiologic changes in older adults make them more susceptible to the potential side effects and toxicities of oral pain medications.
- Interventional pain management techniques that target specific nociceptive transmission sites can reduce pain without the end-organ systemic effects associated with oral pain medications.
- Numerous interventional pain management techniques offer older patients an alternative treatment plan if conservative management is ineffective or contraindicated.

## INTRODUCTION

Chronic pain in older patients is often treated with a combination of pharmacotherapy, physical rehabilitation, interventional pain management, and/or psychological interventions. Pharmacotherapy, or the systemic administration of analgesic medications, is by far the most common treatment. Pain medications are designed to target specific receptors throughout the peripheral and central nervous systems. However, physiologic changes in older adults make them more susceptible to the potential side effects and toxicities of systemically administered pain medications, especially opioids. Interventional pain management is defined as the discipline of medicine devoted to the diagnosis and treatment of pain-related disorders, principally with the application of interventional techniques, independently or in conjunction with other treatment modalities.[1,2] Interventional pain management is a rapidly growing subspecialty.

Disclosure: The authors have nothing to disclose.
[a] Department of Anesthesiology, Wake Forest School of Medicine, Medical Center Boulevard, Winston-Salem, NC 27157-1009, USA; [b] Department of Anesthesiology, Interventional Pain Management, VA Medical Center, Atlanta, GA, USA
* Corresponding author.
*E-mail address:* akbrooks@wakehealth.edu

Interventional pain procedures are performed by a myriad of providers, including, but not limited to, anesthesiologists, physiatrists, neurologists, neurosurgeons, orthopedic surgeons, rheumatologists, and radiologists, all with varying degrees of training. Interventional pain management techniques are designed to target specific nociceptive transmission sites, with the goal of minimizing the intake of oral medications and their end-organ effects. Thus, interventional pain management techniques offer older patients an alternative treatment path with potentially fewer side effects.

This article describes several interventional techniques used to treat the most common sites of pain in older adults: back, knee, and hip.[1] It also reviews data regarding the efficacy and safety of these therapies.

## LUMBAR EPIDURAL INJECTIONS

Lumbar epidural steroid injections (ESIs) are a commonly used procedure for treating a variety of conditions, including lumbar spinal stenosis, lumbar disc herniation, lumbar degenerative disc disease, and lumbosacral radicular pain.[3] An analysis of Medicare use data from 2000 to 2011, showed an increase in epidural and adhesiolysis procedures from a rate of 2172 per 100,000 beneficiaries to 4923 per 100,000 beneficiaries, which represents an increase of 127%.[4] Lumbar spinal stenosis, a common cause of spine-related disability among older adults, is the leading reason for spinal surgery in older adults. Patients with lumbar spinal stenosis report leg pain, lower extremity paresthesia, and/or weakness. Pertinent imaging, including plain films, MRI, and/or computed tomography (CT) scans, should be reviewed before performing an ESI, although there may not be a direct correlation between a patient's symptoms and imaging results. Contraindications to an ESI are listed in **Box 1**.

The lumbar epidural space can be accessed using an interlaminar (midline or paramedian) or transforaminal approach. The transforaminal approach (placement of a needle within the neuroforamen), is used to treat patients with lumbar radicular symptoms who may also have low back pain. Complications of ESIs are described in **Box 2**.[5]

The interlaminar lumbar ESI is performed using fluoroscopic guidance for increased accuracy, as shown in **Fig. 1**. Steroid and/or local anesthetic is injected into the epidural space. There are no clinical trials that examine the ideal number of ESIs. Thus, the number of ESIs should be patient focused and tailored to clinical response.

---

**Box 1**
**Contradictions to epidural steroid injections**

*Absolute contraindications*

- Coagulopathy
- Current anticoagulation use
- Infection: localized near injection site or systemic
- Uncontrolled diabetes mellitus

*Relative contraindications*

- Allergy to medication that will be injected (contrast, local anesthetic, steroid)
- Anatomic changes that would prevent safe procedure (congenital or surgical)
- Immunosuppression

---

**Box 2**
**Complications of epidural steroid injections**

*Drug related*

- Allergy/anaphylaxis to contrast, local anesthetic, steroid
- Local anesthetics: accidental injection into intrathecal space or subdural space could result in hypotension
- Steroids: osteoporosis, avascular necrosis, arachnoiditis, cushingoid symptoms, changes in cognition, irritability, sleep disruption, hyperglycemia, hypertension

*Infection*

- Local skin injection at site of injection, diskitis, epidural abscess, meningitis

*Needle*

- Neural injury from direct needle trauma
- Postdural puncture headache from accidental dural puncture

*Vascular*

- Inadvertent injection of particulate steroid into a vascular structure could lead to ischemia (anterior spinal artery syndrome)

---

There is a considerable amount of controversy surrounding the efficacy of ESIs. The results of clinical trials are heavily influenced by type of specialist (interventional pain specialist vs non–interventional pain specialist), injection (interlaminar vs transforaminal), pain type, and injectate. However, there is general consensus that ESIs provide at least short-term benefit (ie, weeks to months) in well-selected patients.[6] Studies specific to older adults are limited, but most include a wide range of age groups. A recent meta-analysis of 13 randomized controlled trials examined the effects of epidural injections (EIs) with or without steroids in patients with low back pain secondary to lumbar spinal stenosis.[7] Numeric rating scale (NRS) pain scores were available for 10 of

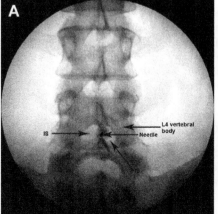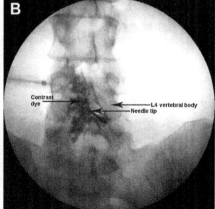

**Fig. 1.** (*A*) Anteroposterior (AP) fluoroscopic image of an interlaminar approach to the L4-5 interspace (IS) using an epidural Tuohy needle. (*B*) AP fluoroscopic image of cephalocaudad spread of contrast dye in the epidural space.

the studies and showed that patients who received steroids in their EIs reported an average reduction of 5.3 (on an 0 to 10 scale) at 3 months, a 4.0 score reduction at 6 months, and a 3.7 score reduction at 12 months. Patients who did not receive steroids in their EIs reported a 4.9 score reduction at 3 months, 4.5 score reduction at 6 months, and a 3.6 reduction at 12 months. There were no significant differences in NRS pain scores between the two groups at 3, 6, or 12 months. There have been few comparative-effectiveness studies comparing ESIs with other treatments. In an underpowered, 6-month, randomized, single-blinded control trial in patients (mean age, 60 years) with lumbar spinal stenosis, both ESIs and physical therapy were effective in reducing pain and improving function for up to 6 months.[8] In conclusion, ESIs seem to provide some short-term pain relief and functional improvement in well-selected patients and should be considered as part of a pain treatment plan for older patients with low back and/or leg pain.

## LUMBAR FACET INJECTIONS

Lumbar facet joints, or zygapophyseal joints, are synovial joints that are innervated by the medial branch (MB) nerves of the dorsal primary ramus. Lumbar facet–mediated pain is a common cause of spinal pain and often associated with functional limitations. Manchikanti and colleagues[9] assessed 100 patients and reported a prevalence of lumbar facet joint–mediated pain confirmed by diagnostic nerve blocks of 52% in patients more than 65 years old and 30% in all adults. Patient-reported low back pain commonly refers to the groin, hip, or thighs, but infrequently below the knee. Increased pain with bending, arching, or twisting movements, and prolonged sitting or standing, is often described. Typical physical examination findings include tenderness over the facet joints and pain with extension and lateral rotation, also known as facet loading. Evidence of lumbar facet arthropathy may also be seen on radiographs, CT scan, or MRI.

Lumbar facet injections are commonly performed. An analysis of Medicare use data from 2000 to 2011 found that lumbar facet injections increased from a rate of 643 per 100,000 in 2000 to a rate of 2111 per 100,000 in 2011. This rate represents a 228% increase in use.[10] Injections for lumbar facet–mediated pain can be performed by injecting directly into the joint or by aiming the injection at the junction of the superior articular process and transverse process (**Fig. 2**) because this is the site where the MB nerve rests. Performing intra-articular facet joint or facet MB joint nerve blocks has long been debated. A 50% reduction in pain after facet MB joint nerve blocks offers the added advantage of proceeding to MB nerve radiofrequency denervation in an attempt to prolong efficacy. A systematic review conducted by Falco and colleagues[11] found improvement in pain with thermal radiofrequency ablation, fair to good evidence to support the use of lumbar facet MB joint nerve blocks, and limited evidence for intra-articular injections.

## PERCUTANEOUS VERTEBRAL AUGMENTATION

It has been estimated that 10 million Americans more than 50 years old have osteoporosis. The rates of osteoporosis are expected to increase by 50% by the year 2025.[12] Vertebral compression fractures (VCFs) are the most common type of fracture secondary to osteoporosis.[12] Only a quarter of VCFs result from falls, and most are precipitated by routine daily activities such as bending or lifting.[13] Osteoporotic VCFs frequently produce a wide range of symptoms, with some patients reporting no pain, whereas others experience significant pain. Of the symptomatic patients, a subset report improvement in their pain with analgesic medications, immobilization

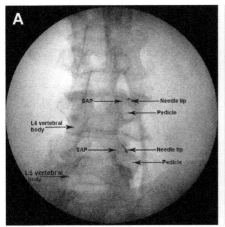
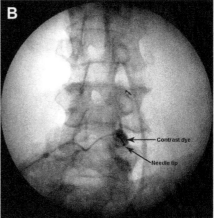

Fig. 2. (*A*) Oblique fluoroscopic image of lumbar facet MB joint nerve block at the L4 and L5 levels. The tip of the needle is located at the junction of the superior articular process (SAP) and the pedicle. (*B*) Contrast dye is used to confirm correct needle placement and lack of intravascular uptake.

therapy via bracing, and physical therapy, whereas others fail conservative management.[14]

Two minimally invasive surgical procedures, vertebroplasty (VP) and kyphoplasty (KP), are commonly used to treat persistent, acute painful fractures. Between 2005 and 2010, 225,259 KPs and 81,790 VPs were performed.[15] In VP, cement is injected percutaneously into the fractured vertebral body via a cannula. Similarly, KP is performed percutaneously, but involves the introduction of a balloon that is inflated in an attempt to restore vertebral body height and create a contained cavity filled with cement (**Fig. 3**). Cement leakage into the spinal canal with resultant neurologic deficits and cement leakage into surrounding vasculature with risk of pulmonary embolism are the most serious complications. Contraindications to VP and KP include existing coagulopathy or use of blood thinners, burst fracture with retropulsed bone, and vertebral height loss greater than 66%.[16]

Two meta-analyses of pooled comparisons of VP and KP versus nonoperative management favored treatment of VCFs with vertebral augmentation. In 2013, Anderson and colleagues[17] reported greater pain relief, functional recovery, and health-related quality of life with vertebral augmentation compared with controls at early (0–3 months) and late (6–12 months) time points. Similarly, Guo and colleagues[18] reported that vertebral augmentation was more effective than nonoperative management in decreasing short-term (0–3 months) and long-term ($\geq$12 months) VCF-associated back pain.

## SACROILIAC JOINT INJECTIONS

The sacroiliac (SI) joints are diarthrodial joints located at the junction of the sacrum and ilium.[19] As humans age, the already small joint space narrows further and becomes filled with debris, making it difficult for it to perform its primary function: absorbing shock from the spine and transmitting it to the pelvis and lower extremities.[20] The SI joint has been implicated as the source of pain in between 13% and 30% of patients with low back pain.[20,21] Older patients are more likely to have SI joint–related low back pain because of decreased ability of the SI joint to absorb shock from the spine.[21]

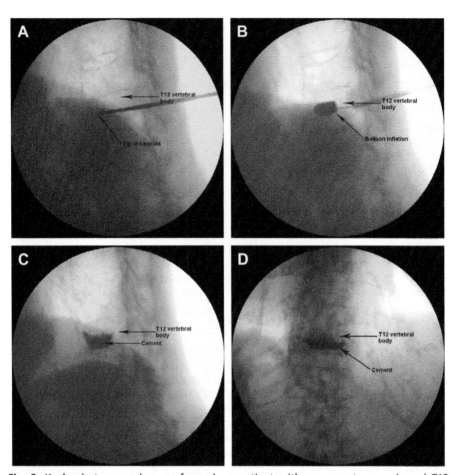

**Fig. 3.** Kyphoplasty procedure performed on patient with severe osteoporosis and T12 vertebral compression fracture. (*A*) Lateral fluoroscopic image of insertion of cannula into the T12 vertebral body. (*B*) Lateral fluoroscopic image of balloon inflation in the T12 vertebral body. (*C*) Lateral fluoroscopic image after removal of the balloon and injection of cement. (*D*) AP fluoroscopic image of vertebral height restoration after injection of cement.

There is no gold standard for diagnosing SI joint pain so it is often a diagnosis of exclusion. Some of the provocative tests commonly used in clinical practice (ie, Faber, distraction, compression, palpation, Gaenslen) do not have high sensitivity or specificity; often 3 or more tests must be performed to increase diagnostic accuracy.[19,21] At times, intra-articular injection with local anesthetic alone is used to confirm the diagnosis.[20] Pain attributable to the SI joint is usually located in the low back area (below the beltline), radiating to the buttocks and posterior thigh, terminating at or just below the knee.[19] Clinically, it is difficult to distinguish SI joint pain from discogenic pain, lumbar myofascial pain, or pain from the lumbar facet joints because SI joint pain may present in the low back, pelvis, buttocks, or sacrum.[19–21]

Conservative measures are considered first-line therapy for patients with SI joint pain. Depending on practitioner or patient preference, these measures may include physical therapy, medication management (muscle relaxants, antiinflammatories), stretching regimens, heat/ice, or transcutaneous electrical nerve stimulation units. If these methods fail to reduce the patient's symptoms, an SI joint steroid injection, usually fluoroscopically guided (**Fig. 4**), is considered. Sacroiliac joint injections are among the fastest growing interventional pain procedures in the United States. A recent analysis of Medicare use data from 2000 to 2011 revealed an increase in SI joint injections from a rate of 125 per 100,000 beneficiaries to 539 per 100,000 beneficiaries, which represents an increase of more than 300%.[22]

With regard to long-term efficacy, the evidence of intra-articular steroid injection is weak at best. The literature features multiple case studies and retrospective analyses/chart reviews reporting the benefits of SI joint injections. At this time, there is no randomized, double-blinded study that compares steroid injections with placebo. A recent meta-analysis concluded that the evidence supporting the efficacy of intra-articular or periarticular injections of local anesthetic or steroids into the SI joint was limited or poor.[23] The best recommendation at this time is to use these injections as adjuncts to a multimodal analgesia regimen with the understanding that it can likely help patients in the short term ($\leq$3 months) but evidence regarding their long-term (>3 months) benefits is lacking.

## OSTEOARTHRITIC JOINT PAIN

Osteoarthritis (OA) is the fastest growing health condition in the United States and is a cause of significant morbidity, economic burden, and decrease in functional status in older adults.[24–27] OA is characterized by degeneration of the articular cartilage and adjacent bone, ligaments, and capsule of the joints that occurs secondary to a combination of genetic predisposition and overloading of the joints.[27–29] According to the Behavioral Risk Factor Surveillance System, 59% of people greater than 65 years of age have arthritis or chronic joint pain.[24] As the proportion of older adults in the general population continues to increase, the number of patients with arthritis or chronic joint pain is expected to increase significantly.[24,26,30,31] Potential complications from polypharmacy, combined with age-related declines in the central nervous, hepatic, and

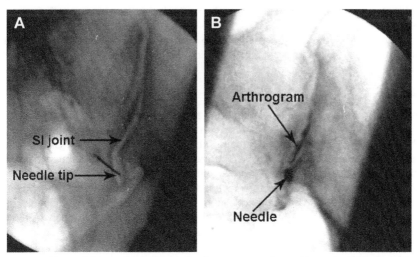

**Fig. 4.** (*A*) Oblique fluoroscopic image of right SI joint with needle tip in view. (*B*) Oblique fluoroscopic image of right SI joint after injection of contrast dye in the joint space (also known as an arthrogram).

renal systems, highlight the necessity for access to nonsurgical, nonpharmacologic options for pain management treatment in older patients.[25]

Interventional pain management for knee and hip OA may be performed using fluoroscopy, MRI, CT scan, ultrasonography (US), or even blind/landmark-based approaches. Within the past decade, there has been a significant increase in the number of US-guided pain procedures. The increased use of US is caused by its reduced risk of radiation exposure to patient and provider, ease of performance, better visualization of the joint of interest (including bony and soft tissue structures), and ability to avoid vascular structures.[32]

In general, 3 types of intra-articular injections may be performed: corticosteroid, hyaluronic acid (HA) (viscosupplementation), and platelet-rich plasma (PRP). These injections are used clinically to manage patients with moderate to severe, symptomatic OA that has not responded favorably to conservative measures such as physical therapy, nonsteroidal antiinflammatory medications, or activity modification. Corticosteroid injections usually contain 40 to 80 mg of a depot steroid preparation such as triamcinolone acetate or methylprednisolone acetate in addition to a local anesthetic such as bupivacaine or lidocaine.

HA is naturally present in the knee joint and functions as a shock absorber and lubricant.[26,27] With OA, the concentration of intra-articular HA and its molecular weight decreases, thereby increasing forces on the joint and decreasing its ability to resist stress.[26,27,31] The most commonly used HA preparations in the United States include Supartz (Smith and Nephew, Memphis, TN), Synvisc (Genzyme Biosurgery, Cambridge, MA), and Orthovisc (Anika Therapeutics, Woburn, MA). These formulations differ in the number of recommended injections (1–5), origin (rooster combs vs bacterial), and molecular weight.[26,27,31]

PRP is the injection of autologous plasma with a high concentration of platelets into an affected joint or other structures of interest.[33] The concerns about use of PRP injections are caused by varied injection techniques, injection schedules, and number of centrifugations of autologous plasma (causing 3-fold to 5-fold difference in platelet content of injectate).[33] PRP injections are thought to relieve OA symptoms via interaction of platelets with intrinsic joint components and the release of growth factors and cytokines by activated platelets, thereby reducing inflammation and promoting healing.[33]

In general, all 3 types of injections are safe and have few side effects. Therefore, the type of injection, frequency, and imaging guidance used are highly dependent on patient factors as well as provider preference.

### Knee Joint

The knee joint is the largest joint in the body and the principal joint affected by OA.[1,32] OA of the knee more commonly affects men (2×) than women and manifests as pain with ambulation, warmth with palpation of the joint, or pain when the joint is moved through its full range of motion.[28,32,34] Progressive OA leads to a reduction in mobility and function, which is associated with significant morbidity in older patients.[1]

Patients are good candidates for injection therapy if they have moderate to severe, recurrent knee pain with imaging consistent with a diagnosis of OA. Knee injections are most commonly performed with US (**Fig. 5**) or fluoroscopic guidance (**Fig. 6**). The injectate of choice may be a combination of local anesthetic and steroids, PRP, or viscosupplements.

In the short term (<3 months), intra-articular injections of corticosteroid and local anesthetic mixtures into the knee joint are more effective than placebo in managing OA-related knee pain with very few side effects or adverse sequelae.[1,31] The

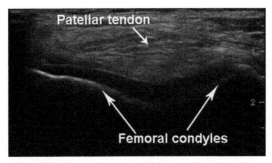

**Fig. 5.** Ultrasonography of the knee joint using a linear US probe. The patellar tendon and femoral condyles are easily viewed.

long-term benefits of steroid injections are not well established. The efficacy of HA injections into the knee joint is also unclear. A recent Cochrane Review of 76 studies that evaluated the efficacy of viscosupplements for the management of knee OA showed that hyaluronates decreased pain and improved function, most notably at the 5-week to 13-week time period after injection.[35] The available meta-analyses are notable for conflicting findings, primarily caused by heterogeneity of the search process and included trials.[27,31] The conclusion is that HA and steroid injections have positive short-term effects that are superior to those of placebo, but their long-term efficacy is still in question.[26,27,31]

At least 2 reviews evaluating the efficacy of PRP injections for knee OA were published in 2015. Meheux and colleagues[36] evaluated 6 articles consisting of 739 patients and concluded that PRP injections improved pain from symptomatic OA for up to 12 months after injection. PRP was also superior to HA in other outcomes, such as pain, physical function, and stiffness over the same time period.[36] Lai and colleagues[37] evaluated 4 articles but their group was unable to come to a conclusion about the relative efficacy of PRP therapy because of small sample sizes and lack of well-designed studies available for analysis.

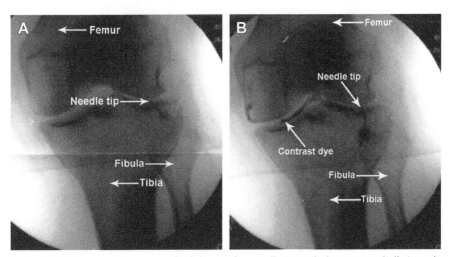

**Fig. 6.** (A) AP fluoroscopic image of left knee. The needle is guided anteromedially into the joint space. (B) AP fluoroscopic image of the left knee after injection of contrast dye in the joint space.

### Hip Joint

The hip joint is a ball and socket joint composed of the articulation of the femoral head with the acetabulum. OA-related hip pain often refers to the groin, low back, and/or buttock and can lead to difficulty with standing or walking. Physical examination usually reveals pain with internal rotation of the hip joint. Older patients who have comorbid conditions that do not make them good surgical candidates for joint replacement or patients wishing to avoid surgical intervention should be considered for injection therapy. In addition, those who have symptoms limiting their daily function or who are unable to use antiinflammatory medications because of history of gastrointestinal bleed or cardiac disease are good candidates for intra-articular hip injections. The most common substance injected into the hip joints is a combination of local anesthetic and steroids. These injections are most often performed using fluoroscopic guidance (**Fig. 7**).

Two recent studies evaluated the efficacy of PRP injections for hip OA.[38,39] Sánchez and colleagues[38] included 40 patients who received 3 PRP injections during the study period. Their pain and functional status were measured at baseline, 6 to 7 weeks, and at the 6-month mark. The results indicated that patients experienced statistically significant reductions in pain (visual analog score, Western Ontario and McMaster Universities Arthritis Index [WOMAC] pain) and improvement in functional status (WOMAC domain for disability) at the end of the 6-month follow-up period.[39] A randomized trial of 100 patients performed by Battaglia and colleagues[40] in 2013 compared the efficacy of US guided intra-articular injections of PRP versus HA for hip OA. At a 12-month follow-up, the investigators reported significant reductions in enrolled patients' pain scores (using the visual analog scale) and improved functional status (as measured by the Harris Hip Score) for the HA and PRP group, with diminishing gains near the end of the 12-month follow-up. PRP was not superior to

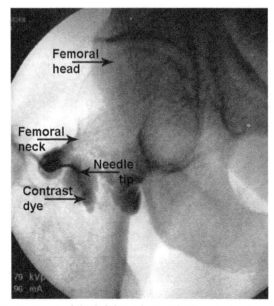

**Fig. 7.** AP fluoroscopic image of the left hip. The needle is passed just medial to the femoral artery until the joint capsule is pierced. Contrast dye is injected to ensure that the spread is intra-articular.

hyaluronate injections in relieving pain from hip OA in this study. Significant limitations in both studies were small sample sizes, variable injection volume, platelet content, and injection schedules.

## SUMMARY

When treating chronic pain in older patients, clinicians must consider the physiology of aging and its effects on the clinical aspects of analgesic interventions. Older patients are more susceptible to the potential side effects of oral pain medications, especially opioids. A variety of interventional pain management techniques offer an alternative treatment plan to failed conservative management or perhaps a large surgical procedure. However, further study is needed to identify when in the pain course an older patient is likely to benefit from a pain specialist's expertise. The procedures are performed using image guidance to increase accuracy and efficiency. Lumbar ESIs in elderly patients with lumbar spinal stenosis who have back pain with or without radicular symptoms are likely to achieve treatment benefit in the short term; however, additional clinical trials focused on this population are needed to further determine their long-term effectiveness. Lumbar facet MB joint radiofrequency denervation offers patients who have responded favorably to diagnostic lumbar facet MB joint injections additional pain relief. Vertebral augmentation via KP and VP is a minimally invasive procedure that could allow patients with severe, refractory back pain to return to their activities of daily living with measurable improvements in their pain. In addition, PRP holds promise for treating end-stage OA, but additional well-powered clinical trials assessing long-term benefit are necessary.

## REFERENCES

1. Abdulla A, Adams N, Bone M, et al. Guidance on the management of pain in older people. Age Ageing 2013;42(Suppl 1):i1–57.
2. Manchikanti L, Boswell MV, Raj PP, et al. Evolution of interventional pain management. Pain Physician 2003;6:485–94.
3. Abraham NR, Badiola I, Vo TD. Epidural (cervical, thoracic, lumbar, caudal) block/injections. In: Deer TR, Leong MS, editors. Treatment of chronic pain by interventional approaches. The American Academy of Pain Medicine textbook on pain medicine. New York: Springer; 2014. p. 149–57.
4. Manchikanti L, Falco FJ, Singh V, et al. Utilization of interventional techniques in managing chronic pain in the Medicare population: analysis of growth patterns from 2000 to 2011. Pain Physician 2012;15:E969–82.
5. McGrath JM, Schaefer MP, Malkamaki DM. Incidence and characteristics of complications from epidural steroid injections. Pain Med 2011;12:726–31.
6. Cohen SP, Bicket MC, Jamison D, et al. Epidural steroids: a comprehensive, evidence-based review. Reg Anesth Pain Med 2013;38:175–200.
7. Meng H, Fei Q, Wang B, et al. Epidural injections with or without steroids in managing chronic low back pain secondary to lumbar spinal stenosis: a meta-analysis of 13 randomized controlled trials. Drug Des Devel Ther 2015;9:4657–67.
8. Koc Z, Ozcakir S, Sivrioglu K, et al. Effectiveness of physical therapy and epidural steroid injections in lumbar spinal stenosis. Spine (Phila Pa 1976) 2009;34:985–9.
9. Manchikanti L, Pampati V, Rivera J, et al. Role of facet joints in chronic low back pain in the elderly: a controlled comparative prevalence study. Pain Pract 2001;1:332–7.

10. Manchikanti L, Pampati V, Singh V, et al. Assessment of the escalating growth of facet joint interventions in the Medicare population in the United States from 2000 to 2011. Pain Physician 2013;16:E365–78.

11. Falco FJ, Manchikanti L, Datta S, et al. An update of the effectiveness of therapeutic lumbar facet joint interventions. Pain Physician 2012;15:E909–53.

12. Burge R, Dawson-Hughes B, Solomon DH, et al. Incidence and economic burden of osteoporosis-related fractures in the United States, 2005-2025. J Bone Miner Res 2007;22:465–75.

13. Holroyd C, Cooper C, Dennison E. Epidemiology of osteoporosis. Best Pract Res Clin Endocrinol Metab 2008;22:671–85.

14. Alexandru D, So W. Evaluation and management of vertebral compression fractures. Perm J 2012;16:46–51.

15. Goz V, Errico TJ, Weinreb JH, et al. Vertebroplasty and kyphoplasty: national outcomes and trends in utilization from 2005 through 2010. Spine J 2015;15:959–65.

16. Truumees E, Hilibrand A, Vaccaro AR. Percutaneous vertebral augmentation. Spine J 2004;4:218–29.

17. Anderson PA, Froyshteter AB, Tontz WL Jr. Meta-analysis of vertebral augmentation compared with conservative management for osteoporotic spinal fractures. J Bone Miner Res 2013;28:372–82.

18. Guo JB, Zhu Y, Chen BL, et al. Surgical versus non-surgical treatment for vertebral compression fracture with osteopenia: a systematic review and meta-analysis. PLoS One 2015;10:e0127145.

19. Rathmell JP. Sacroiliac joint injection. In: Atlas of image-guided spine intervention in regional anesthesia and pain medicine. 1st edition. Philadelphia: Lippincott Williams & Wilkins; 2006. p. 93–100.

20. Foley BS, Buschbacher RM. Sacroiliac joint pain: anatomy, biomechanics, diagnosis, and treatment. Am J Phys Med Rehabil 2006;85:997–1006.

21. Cohen SP, Chen Y, Neufeld NJ. Sacroiliac joint pain: a comprehensive review of epidemiology, diagnosis and treatment. Expert Rev Neurother 2013;13:99–116.

22. Manchikanti L, Hansen H, Pampati V, et al. Utilization and growth patterns of sacroiliac joint injections from 2000 to 2011 in the Medicare population. Pain Physician 2013;16:E379–90.

23. Hansen H, Manchikanti L, Simopoulos TT, et al. A systematic evaluation of the therapeutic effectiveness of sacroiliac joint interventions. Pain Physician 2012; 15:E247–78.

24. Leveille SG. Musculoskeletal aging. Curr Opin Rheumatol 2004;16:114–8.

25. Kaye AD, Baluch A, Scott JT. Pain management in the elderly population: a review. Ochsner J 2010;10:179–87.

26. Benke M, Shaffer B. Viscosupplementation treatment of arthritis pain. Curr Pain Headache Rep 2009;13:440–6.

27. Hunter DJ. Viscosupplementation for osteoarthritis of the knee. N Engl J Med 2015;372:1040–7.

28. Sinusas K. Osteoarthritis: diagnosis and treatment. Am Fam Physician 2012;85: 49–56.

29. Millett PJ, Gobezie R, Boykin RE. Shoulder osteoarthritis: diagnosis and management. Am Fam Physician 2008;78:605–11.

30. Centers for Disease Control and Prevention (CDC). Public health and aging: projected prevalence of self-reported arthritis or chronic joint symptoms among persons aged >65 years–United States, 2005-2030. MMWR Morb Mortal Wkly Rep 2003;52:489–91.

31. Reid MC. Viscosupplementation for osteoarthritis: a primer for primary care physicians. Adv Ther 2013;30:967–86.
32. Korbe S, Udoji EN, Ness TJ, et al. Ultrasound-guided interventional procedures for chronic pain management. Pain Manag 2015;5:466–82.
33. Ornetti P, Nourissat G, Berenbaum F, et al. Does platelet-rich plasma have a role in the treatment of osteoarthritis? Joint Bone Spine 2016;83(1):31–6.
34. Narouze S, Raju SVY. Joint injections. In: Benzon HT, Raja SN, Liu SS, et al, editors. Essentials of pain medicine. 3rd edition. Philadelphia: Saunders; 2011. p. 423–30.
35. Bellamy N, Campbell J, Robinson V, et al. Viscosupplementation for the treatment of osteoarthritis of the knee. Cochrane Database Syst Rev 2006;(2):CD005321.
36. Meheux CJ, McCulloch PC, Lintner DM, et al. Efficacy of intra-articular platelet-rich plasma injections in knee osteoarthritis: a systematic review. Arthroscopy 2016;32(3):495–505.
37. Lai LP, Stitik TP, Foye PM, et al. Use of platelet-rich plasma in intra-articular knee injections for osteoarthritis: a systematic review. PM R 2015;7:637–48.
38. Sánchez M, Guadilla J, Fiz N, et al. Ultrasound-guided platelet-rich plasma injections for the treatment of osteoarthritis of the hip. Rheumatology (Oxford) 2012; 51:144–50.
39. Battaglia M, Guaraldi F, Vannini F, et al. Platelet-rich plasma (PRP) intra-articular ultrasound-guided injections as a possible treatment for hip osteoarthritis: a pilot study. Clin Exp Rheumatol 2011;29:754.
40. Battaglia M, Guaraldi F, Vannini F, et al. Efficacy of ultrasound-guided intra-articular injections of platelet-rich plasma versus hyaluronic acid for hip osteoarthritis. Orthopedics 2013;36:e1501–8.

# Role of Emerging Technologies in Geriatric Pain Management

Rachael Elizabeth Docking, PhD

## KEYWORDS

- Older adults • Technology • Pain management • Pain assessment • Apps
- mHealth

## KEY POINTS

- Emerging technologies can help to create innovative methods to assess and manage in older adults.
- Although there is some evidence for the efficacy of the technologies, existing studies rarely focus on older populations.
- There are still several changes required to ensure the secure use of technology in clinical settings; for example, acute care, long-term care, urgent care, and primary care.
- Most pain applications that have been developed so far have had almost no input from health care professionals or end users. Future technologies should be developed with appropriate clinical and end user partners to maximize their relevance.

## INTRODUCTION

The use of technology has become a key part of life as the availability of tablets and smartphones has continued to increase. Innovation has moved to focus on emerging new technologies and their ability to improve health and wellbeing. In particular, applications (apps) can be used by consumers and patients as part of homecare and self-care, thus potentially providing cost savings to health systems.[1] As pointed out by the recent report from the IMS Institute for Healthcare Informatics, although there is increasing enthusiasm for the use of technology in health care, the use of apps still remains a novelty.

The past century has seen an increase in life expectancy[2] and, for the first time, people 60 years and older outnumber those younger than 16 years.[3] With increasing age comes the increase of diseases of old age such as dementia, arthritis, and cancer. Dementia affects approximately 35.6 million persons globally[4] and it has been estimated

Faculty of Health, Social Care and Education, Anglia Ruskin University, London, 4th Floor William Harvey Building, Bishop Hall Lane, Chelmsford Essex, CM1 1SQ, UK
*E-mail address:* rachael.docking@anglia.ac.uk

Clin Geriatr Med 32 (2016) 787–795
http://dx.doi.org/10.1016/j.cger.2016.06.011     **geriatric.theclinics.com**
0749-0690/16/Crown Copyright © 2016 Published by Elsevier Inc. All rights reserved.

that the prevalence of dementia will double every 20 years (Ferri and colleagues,[5] 2005). There is also evidence that the prevalence of pain increases with age, particularly disabling pain or pain sufficient to interfere with day-to-day living.[6–8] Dionne and colleagues[6] reviewed epidemiologic studies that examined back pain prevalence by age and found that although older people experience a decrease in nondisabling back pain they experience an increased prevalence of disabling back pain. Docking and colleagues[8] found, in a United Kingdom (UK) population, that although nondisabling back pain plateaued in older age, disabling back pain continued to increase in the oldest old. Also, Thomas and colleagues[7] reported that the onset of pain that interferes with everyday life continues to increase with age.

This increase in pain in older adults, along with the increasing use of technology, presents a huge opportunity for health care staff and researchers to harness advances in technology to develop new ways of assessing pain and delivering education, support, and behavior change interventions for the management of pain in later life.[9] Due to the increased use of technology within health care, the World Health Organization (WHO) has coined the term mobile health (mHealth), which refers to medical and public health practice supported by mobile devices.[10]

Certain patient groups have greater challenges and barriers to accessing care (eg, older adults) due to problems such as geographic distance from health care centers, obtaining transportation services, and increased mobility difficulties. Therefore, the use of technology-based approaches for older people with various pain conditions may lead to significant cost savings in intervention delivery but also improved quality of life and feelings of control among patients.

The demand for support for pain management and assessment in older adults is set to grow rapidly as the population continues to age. There is a need for sufficient evidence of the benefit technology can offer regarding improved patient outcomes and reduced health care costs. Additionally, those in the health and care services will need to embrace more technology-enabled products, services, and systems to allow for the successful and efficient management of pain in the older population. This article provides a brief overview of the challenges and opportunities that technology can offer geriatric pain management and reviews emerging evidence to demonstrate the role that technology can play in improving and advancing how to not only assess but manage pain in older adults.

## EVIDENCE REGARDING THE USE OF TECHNOLOGY FOR PAIN CARE

The last few years have seen substantial progress in ways to make the management of pain as accurate, reliable, and convenient as possible, including technology-assisted self-management interventions, electronic pain diaries, clinical dashboards, and interventions delivered using Internet and mobile apps. The following section discusses some of the evidence regarding the use of technology for assessing and managing pain among older adults.

### Pain Assessment

Currently, there is limited research to inform the assessment and management of pain in those 65 years of age and older, particularly those with dementia. Evidence suggests that this group may not receive adequate assessment of their pain[11] and pain that is assessed is often undertreated or poorly managed.[12–14] One innovative example of how technology could help to improve the assessment of pain in older adults with dementia is described in the following section.

### *Evaluation of the iPhone Pain Assessment Application for People with Dementia*

Given the aging of the population, greater numbers of older adults are living in their own homes and will require the use of emergency (eg, paramedic) services. Pain management in the paramedic setting is increasingly important in the UK ambulance services where 80% of patients present with pain-related complaints (in other countries as well).[15,16] Paramedics report barriers to providing adequate pain relief such as concerns about patient accuracy in evaluating their own pain and the effect of analgesia interfering with clinical assessments. Furthermore, paramedics identified that many patients with dementia or cognitive impairments have problems communicating their pain and, as such, pain may be ignored, overlooked, or mistaken for challenging behavior.[15] Currently, national clinical guidelines for paramedics recommend the Verbal Rating Score and Wong-Baker FACES Scale to assess pain. However, these scales do not account for patients who have difficulty communicating.

Considering this, researchers at the University of Greenwich collaborated with the Computing and Mathematical Sciences department to develop an iPhone pain assessment app (**Fig. 1**).

This app was evaluated in the South London Ambulance Service (LAS) National Health Service (NHS) Trust and the South East Coast Ambulance (SECAmb) Service NHS Foundation Trust to explore the feasibility of using it to assess pain among adults with dementia in the paramedic setting and to explore paramedic students' ideas on how the app could be modified or improved.[17] Following this, recommended changes put forward by the paramedic students were presented to an expert panel of paramedics who selected those most relevant for future implementation of the app.

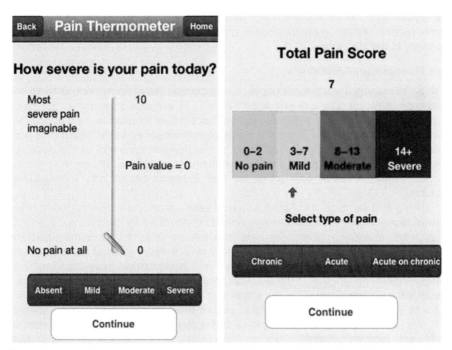

**Fig. 1.** iPhone pain assessment app screenshots. (*Courtesy of* University of Greenwich, London, United Kingdom; with permission.)

The results indicated that the iPhone pain assessment tool for older adults with cognitive impairment could be a useful tool in the prehospital setting and, potentially, other populations with communication difficulties. Evidence suggests that one of the most common reasons for dialing 999 (911 in the US) is because an individual is experiencing pain.[18] Providing access to a tool in the paramedic setting that has been specifically developed to help identify and assess pain in a user-friendly format may well result in improvements in pain management and, subsequently, improved quality of life for the adult with dementia.

The most common concerns raised, however, were the use of technology in the clinical setting and how appropriate it is to use electronic devices while working with a patient, as well as the lack of adequate support for paramedic staff to allow them the opportunity to use app-based assessment methods in practice. Most participants did not think that use of an iPad, or similar electronic device, was currently possible in the clinical setting.

The development of apps such as this provides new insights into innovative methods for pain assessment for older adults, particularly those with cognitive impairment. The benefits of implementing such a tool are potentially wide reaching, improving health care professionals' knowledge and confidence in pain assessment for older adults, thereby improving pain management. In addition, there is huge potential for wider application of the tool along with national implementation in the paramedic emergency service system. Other possible clinical situations in which the app could be used include emergency departments, acute care wards, and nursing homes. There is also the potential for use within an informal care setting.

### Pain Management

A recent report from the Institute of Medicine recommended the promotion of self-management of pain through the use of technology.[19] The following section describes some recent technology-related pain management techniques that have been reviewed in the literature.

### Pain Management Applications

With an increasing use of smartphones, it is becoming increasingly popular to download apps. A recent review of pain apps[20] found 111 available apps across the major mobile platforms. The investigators included apps if they focused on pain education, pain management, or pain relief, and were not specifically aimed at health care professionals. There was limited health care professional involvement in the development of the apps (86% reported no involvement). All pain apps offered the promise of pain relief; however, few contained any evidence-based pain management features.

Palermo and Jamison[9] published a special series providing a contemporary overview of technology-assisted self-management interventions for chronic pain in adults. They were examining patient-focused smartphone apps for pain management. Palermo and Jamison[9] rated the functionality of 279 apps, most of these provided self-monitoring or pain education; however, few implemented more than one pain self-management function. Further, most were designed without any input from health care professionals. The investigators concluded that it is essential for pain apps to include input from scientists to ensure they are robust and valid. Palermo and Jamison[9] thought that the topic of technology and pain self-management is timely and they encouraged future research in this area. Potential benefits include improved pain management for the individual but also a significant reduction in the economic cost of chronic pain. Of note, the evidence summarized in the review focused on children, adolescents, and adults; none of the reviewed studies focused on older adults.

A recent review by the IMS Institute for Healthcare Informatics[1] reported on a whole range of health care apps, some of which related to pain management in the adult population, but none specific to older adults. For example, the WebMD pain coach is an app that provides a holistic approach to balancing lifestyle with chronic pain conditions. WebMD is designed as a mobile companion, allowing patients to be in control of their lifestyle choices and to review personal patterns to understand triggers, set goals, and easily share progress with health care staff. The only other pain-related app reviewed within this report was Zimmer Arthritis 411, which is a patient education resource for people who suffer from arthritis. It is designed to be used either by the patient or in conjunction with the clinician during consultation. These have not been further reviewed or validated so it is not possible to report on their effectiveness in improving pain management in older adults.

### Clinical Dashboards

A clinical dashboard is a tool that aims to provide clinicians with relevant information. They provide clinicians with quick and easy access to health care data that are being captured locally, along with information to help them make clinical decisions, such as best practice advice.

Anderson and colleagues[21] evaluated the impact of a clinical dashboard for opioid analgesic management on opioid prescribing and adherence to opioid practice guidelines in primary care. They evaluated electronic health record data from patients receiving chronic opioid therapy. After implementation of the dashboard, there was an increased adherence to certain opioid practice guidelines, including rate of urine drug testing, signing an opioid treatment agreement, conducting assessment of pain-related functional status, and having at least one visit with a behavioral health provider. There was also some evidence of a decline in chronic opioid therapy.

### Internet-Based Interventions

A recent review by Bender and colleagues[22] examined articles published between 1990 and 2010 that evaluated evidence for Internet-based interventions for individuals with chronic pain. The review found that the interventions consisted mainly of (1) cognitive behavioral therapy (CBT), (2) moderated peer-support programs, or (3) clinical support interventions. The Internet CBT interventions were predominantly structured, self-administered programs that provided minimal support from health care staff. Peer support programs were those that allowed people with similar symptoms to exchange experiences and use a network of support. Whereas clinical support interventions were those that, for example, allowed the patient to access educational Web sites to prepare for doctor visits and provide self-management advice afterward. Most CBT interventions for pain management demonstrated an improvement in pain, improved function, and decreased costs compared with standard care. However, the effects on depression and anxiety were less consistent, which may be due to the lack of person contact. The online peer-support network evidence showed a significant reduction in the prevalence of pain and anxiety, and reduced loneliness and withdrawn behavior. Finally, clinical support interventions helped to significantly reduce pain and improved patient's knowledge. Although this evidence was interesting, there was no specific focus on older adults, with most of the evidence focusing on children and young adults.

### Text Messaging

There is currently limited evidence regarding the effectiveness of text messaging for pain management and nothing specific to older adults. Recent evidence published in 2015[23] examined the preliminary effectiveness of a text message–based social support intervention for adults that aimed to reduce daily pain and pain interference, improve affect and perceptions of social support in patients with chronic noncancer pain, and explore the feasibility of a novel mobile app to track perceptions of pain and pain interference. Results found modest reductions in pain in those who received the text messages. Although this study was not specific to older adults, it did include older adults within the sample and provides some support for the feasibility of such methods in improving patients' daily experience of pain.

A recent review summarizes existing evidence regarding the compliance, feasibility, user-friendliness, reliability, and validity of text messaging in pain patients.[10] Text messages could be an inexpensive way for communication between patients and health care professionals for chronic pain management. Further, this method could be easily integrated into mobiles or smartphones, which most of the population own.

## CHALLENGES WITH TECHNOLOGY
### Challenges for Health Care Staff Using Technology for Pain Management

The recent evaluation of the iPhone pain assessment app by Docking and colleagues,[17] previously described, uncovered a range of challenges that health care professionals might face when using technology in the clinical setting. These challenges are detailed briefly in the following section.

### Appropriateness of Technology in the Clinical Setting

There are questions around the appropriateness of using technology within the clinical setting and the lack of adequate support for clinical staff to allow them the opportunity to use app-based methods in practice. In the evaluation of the iPhone pain app, most participants did not think that use of an electronic device was currently feasible in the clinical setting. This was predominantly due to their worries over perceptions of patients while using such devices. Suggestions to address this barrier include using current electronic systems in which the app could be incorporated, and changing the way in which clinicians work and record data to a more electronic-based method. All participants were in agreement that as the technology age advances there will be an increased need for technology in the clinical setting that will bring with it greater acceptance and understanding from patients of the benefit such methods can bring.

### Cost

There is a clear need for a cost analysis regarding the effectiveness of technology-based interventions. Taking into account the development and maintenance costs, savings across the health care system must be demonstrated and there is currently a lack of cost-analysis studies to show this outcome.

Health care systems have recently made a move toward the use of electronic health records. Therefore, it might be feasible to allow for an integration of mobile app-generated data into these systems, which could potentially reduce costs. However, this will require a huge amount of collaboration between stakeholders to allow for a smooth transition into a new technology-led health care system.

## Infrastructure

The infrastructure required for a move toward technology does not currently exist from both a health care and a patient perspective. There are serious concerns around data privacy and security when using such methods. It is therefore essential that it is clear how data within apps will be used, ensuring patient consent is provided, and that the information held is secure, particularly if there is integration with electronic health records and health-related apps. With the potential for confidential patient information to be passed between systems, it is essential this is done in a secure manner and, currently, there is no infrastructure to support that.

## Technical Support

Current apps are not yet compatible with hospital-based electronic medical records and, as a result, there will be issues with data transfer. It is unclear who would have the responsibility to provide technical support for apps: medical informaticians, app providers, or both. Although apps should save time and money and reduce face-to-face visits, there could be additional costs if technical problems occur and regularly persist.

## Hygiene

When using apps in the clinical setting, it is essential to be aware of the spread of infections. If tools, such as tablets, are used for pain assessment and management in a clinic, it is important that these are given suitable covers that can be regularly cleaned if they are used across patients.

## Challenges for Patients Using Technology for Pain Management

There is currently limited evidence to help patients understand the apps that are currently available and which apps might be most useful in assisting patients with the task of self-managing pain. This is a particular challenge for older adults who may have limited online experience and be less able to research the evidence base for health-related apps. Older adults may also not feel comfortable using certain software, and there may be challenges around reading, language, or cognitive skills.[9]

In the UK, the NHS developed and launched a library of NHS-reviewed apps (in 2013) aimed at empowering people to manage their own health. The NHS reviewed apps available on the market to provide consumers with evidence of which apps were clinically safe and reliable. With increasing health care costs and limited funding, the library was designed to encourage patients to be active participants in how their health is managed. Although this Web site was a step in the right direction, it did not answer all the concerns around the use of apps in health care, particularly in relation to security of patient information. The library has now been closed after coming to the end of a period of testing. However, there are plans to conduct an evaluation, glean any lessons that can be learned from this initiative, and help to inform the development of something similar in the future. Concerns over the safety and security of patient information, however, have been raised. A recent study[24] found that many of the apps that were recommended failed to provide adequate protection of patient data. The investigators reported that out of 35 apps in the library that sent identifying information over the Internet, 23 did so without encryption. Therefore, although such a library would be welcomed, steps need to be taken to address these concerns and make changes where needed.

## SUMMARY

Technology has the potential to play an instrumental role in serving patients by making health care more affordable, accessible, and available. Although the future role of technology in the management of pain in the older population is promising, there are clearly current challenges that need to be addressed before technology can be fully integrated into the health care system.

mHealth might provide us with the opportunity to collect clinical, patient lifestyle, and behavior data, which could improve communication between the patient and the health care provider, and may also aid in the assessment of pain within the clinical setting. However, few technologies currently exist to meet the needs of older people with chronic pain.

In addition, there is limited evidence that the technology leads to improved patient outcomes or reduces use of health care services.[10] Further work is needed to look into the impact of apps on hospital and clinic visits before additional money is spent developing and testing new innovations, as well as to clarify whether technology can ultimately contribute to a reduction in the burden of chronic pain.

With further evidence and input from health care professionals and patients on what they actually need from emerging technologies, it might be possible to take advantage of what the technology age has to offer, to develop and use tools that can potentially improve the quality of life for older adults living with pain, and to ensure they can remain living independently and within their own homes for as long as possible.

Author's key recommendations

- With currently limited technologies that meet the needs of older people with chronic pain and questions around improved outcomes from technology, there is currently not enough evidence to recommend that health care professionals make use of current pain apps.
- However, as technology develops within this field, health care professionals should remain up to date on evidence as it emerges.
- The recently closed NHS library of NHS-reviewed apps is potentially going to reopen following its initial pilot testing phase. If this does happen, this would be an ideal place for health care professionals to start if interested in using apps within their practice, to identify the most useful and well-evaluated apps available for pain management.

## REFERENCES

1. Aitken M, Gauntlett C. Patient apps for improved healthcare: from novelty to mainstream. Parsippany (NJ): IMS Institute for Healthcare Informatics; 2013.
2. Tse MMY, Pun SPY, Benzie IFF. Pain relief strategies used by older people with chronic pain: an exploratory survey for planning patient-centred intervention. J Clin Nurs 2005;14(3):315–20.
3. Office of National Statistics. 2010. Available at: http://www.statistics.gov.uk/default.asp. Accessed December 4, 2015.
4. World Health Organisation. Dementia: a public health priority. United Kingdom: Alzheimer's Disease International; 2012. Available at: http://www.who.int/mental_health/publications/dementia_report_2012/en/. Accessed July 8, 2015.
5. Ferri CP, Prince M, Brayne C, et al. Global prevalence of dementia: a Delphi consensus study. Lancet 2005;366(9503):2112–7.
6. Dionne CE, Dunn KM, Croft PR. Does back pain prevalence really decrease with increasing age? A systematic review. Age Ageing 2005;35(3):229–34.

7. Thomas E, Mottram S, Peat G, et al. The effect of age on the onset of pain interference in a general population of older adults: prospective findings from the North Staffordshire Osteoarthritis Project (NorStOP). Pain 2007;129:21–7.
8. Docking RE, Fleming J, Brayne C, et al, Cambridge City over-75s Cohort Study Collaboration. Epidemiology of back pain in older adults: prevalence and risk factors for back pain onset. Rheumatology (Oxford) 2011;50(9):1645–53.
9. Palermo TM, Jamison RN. Innovative delivery of pain management interventions: current trends and future progress. Clin J Pain 2015;31(6):467–9.
10. Vardeh D, Edwards RR, Jamison RN, et al. There's an app for that: mobile technology is a new advantage in managing chronic pain. ISAP Pain Clinical Updates 2013;21(6):1–7.
11. Closs SJ, Barr B, Briggs M, et al. A comparison of five pain assessment scales for nursing home residents with varying degrees of cognitive impairment. J Pain Symptom Manage 2004;27(3):196–205.
12. Helme RD, Gibson SJ. Pain in older people. In: Crombie IK, Croft PR, Linton SJ, et al, editors. Epidemiology of pain. Seattle (WA): IASP Press; 1999. p. 103–12.
13. Scherder E, Oosterman J, Swaab D, et al. Recent developments in pain in dementia. Br Med J 2005;330(7489):461–4.
14. Williams E, Sutton S. Elderly fallers referrals: update. United Kingdom: London Ambulance Service; 2012. Clin Update 28. Available at: http://www.londonambulance.nhs.uk/health_professionals/gp_information/idoc.ashx?docid=c5ec9929-66a8-41a1-8e9a-28d08fe25278&version=-1. Accessed December 4, 2015.
15. Harvey C. Is there scope for an observational pain scoring tool in paramedic practice? J Paramedic Pract 2014;6(2):84–8.
16. Bonica JJ, Loeser JJ, Chapman CR, et al. The management of pain. Philadelphia: Lea and Febiger; 1990.
17. Docking RE, Lane M, Schofield PA. Developing an iPhone APP for the assessment of pain in older adults with dementia. Presented at the 7th International Congress of Pain in Dementia, Bergen, Norway, April 24–25, 2015.
18. McLean SA, Maio RF, Domeier RM. The epidemiology of pain in the prehospital setting. Prehosp Emerg Care 2002;6(4):402–5.
19. Simon LS. Relieving pain in America: a blueprint for transforming prevention, care, education, and research. Journal of Pain & Palliative Care Pharmacotherapy 2012;26(2):197–8.
20. Rosser BA, Eccleston C. Smartphone applications for pain management. J Telemed Telecare 2011;17(6):308–12.
21. Anderson D, Zlateva I, Khatri K, et al. Using health information technology to improve adherence to opioid prescribing guidelines in primary care. Clin J Pain 2015;31(6):573.
22. Bender JL, Radhakrishnan A, Diorio C, et al. Can pain be managed through the Internet? A systematic review of randomized controlled trials. Pain 2011;152(8):1740–50.
23. Guillory J, Chang P, Henderson CR Jr, et al. Piloting a text message–based social support intervention for patients with chronic pain: establishing feasibility and preliminary efficacy. Clin J Pain 2015;31(6):548–56.
24. Huckvale K, Prieto JT, Tilney M, et al. Unaddressed privacy risks in accredited health and wellness apps: a cross-sectional systematic assessment. BMC Med 2015;13(1):214.

# Expanding Targets for Intervention in Later Life Pain

## What Role Can Patient Beliefs, Expectations, and Pleasant Activities Play?

M. Carrington Reid, MD, PhD

### KEYWORDS

- Beliefs and attitudes • Patient expectations • Pleasant activity scheduling

### KEY POINTS

- Certain pain beliefs and attitudes negatively affect older adults' willingness to engage in and/or adhere with treatment, can adversely impact treatment outcomes, and are amenable to change. Clinicians should assess older patients' beliefs and attitudes prior to initiating treatment.
- Patient expectations can impact treatment outcomes and are potentially malleable. Clinicians caring for older adults with chronic pain should routinely assess patients' treatment expectancies (eg, degree of pain relief expected and the degree of functional improvement the patient hopes to achieve) prior to initiating treatment.
- Pleasurable activity restriction is common in older patients with chronic pain and constitutes an important target for intervention. Clinicians should include pleasant activity scheduling as part of their multimodal treatment plan, particularly for those patients who endorse cutting back or eliminating pleasurable activities.

Pain is one of the most common conditions health care providers encounter when caring for older patients. Treating pain in older patients is challenging because of a variety of physical (eg, age-related physiologic changes; onset of sensory and cognitive impairments or gait and balance problems; and multimorbidity and associated polypharmacy) and psychosocial (eg, affective disorders, care-rejecting behaviors, or social isolation) factors that constrain treatment choices.[1] A limited evidence base to guide treatment also constitutes a significant barrier to effective geriatric pain management.[2] Pain generators such as spinal stenosis or advanced osteoarthritis often can not be

Disclosures: The author has nothing to disclose.
Division of Geriatrics and Palliative Medicine, Weill Cornell Medicine, 525 East 68th Street, #39, New York, NY 10065, USA
E-mail address: mcr2004@med.cornell.edu

Clin Geriatr Med 32 (2016) 797–805
http://dx.doi.org/10.1016/j.cger.2016.06.009
0749-0690/16/© 2016 Elsevier Inc. All rights reserved.

**geriatric.theclinics.com**

targeted because of the factors noted previously or because of patient concerns about undergoing a surgical procedure.

As described in previous articles in this series, targets for intervention include

1. Pain reduction using pharmacotherapies (see Jennifer Greene Naples, Walid F. Gellad, Joseph T. Hanlon's article, "The Role of Opioid Analgesics in Geriatric Pain Management" and Zachary A. Marcum, Nakia A. Duncan, Una E. Makris's article, "Pharmacotherapies in Geriatric Chronic Pain Management," in this issue), interventional approaches that do not involve surgery (see Amber K. Brooks, Mercy A. Udoji's article, "Interventional Techniques for Management of Pain in Older Adults," in this issue) and/or non-drug therapies,
2. Preservation of function by means of exercise and other physical therapies (see Sean Laubenstein, Katherine Beissner's article, "Exercise and Movement-Based Therapies in Geriatric Pain Management," in this issue), and
3. Coping skills training as a way of helping patients to adapt to pain and its consequences (see Christopher Eccleston, Abby Tabor, Rhiannon Terri Edwards, and Edmund Keogh's article, "Psychological Approaches to Coping with Pain in Later Life," in this issue).

Augmenting the number and type of targets clinicians have at their disposal is important to do. These targets can be factors that amplify the adverse effects of pain or mediate its effects and help providers to broaden their portfolio of pain management options. For example, among patients with depressed mood and pain, clinicians often direct treatment at the depressive symptoms, particularly when the patient cannot be prescribed (or tolerate) a pain medication, achieving positive results in the form of reduced depressive symptomatology and pain. Similarly, targeting sleep problems in patients with comorbid pain and sleep disturbance often leads to reduced pain and improved functioning.

This article highlights 3 additional targets clinicians should consider when initiating treatment plans for older patients with chronic pain: (1) patient attitudes and beliefs about pain and pain treatments, (2) patient expectations regarding treatment outcomes, and (3) pleasurable activity scheduling. Evidence supporting these recommendations is provided, as well as practical strategies to intervene on each in the outpatient setting.

## PAIN ATTITUDES AND BELIEFS

Older adults can maintain attitudes and beliefs about pain and pain treatments that negatively influence expectations regarding treatment outcome, impact specific health behaviors, and negatively affect their willingness to engage in and/or adhere with specific treatments. Many theories of health behavior (eg, social cognitive theory) highlight the important role that patients' attitudes (a settled way of thinking or feeling about something) and beliefs (a feeling or thought that something is true) play regarding behaviors such as engaging in physical activity or taking a prescribed medication as directed.[3] Patient attitudes and beliefs about pain and specific pain treatments come from varied sources, including friends and other members of their social network, family, social media, patients' health care providers, and their own experiences living with chronic pain, often over many years.

What types of pain-related beliefs and attitudes do older adults endorse, and how common are they? In 1 survey of community-dwelling older adults, more than 50% of participants considered arthritis-related pain to be a natural part of getting old.[4] In a large study of veterans, those who were older (65 and above) were far more likely to believe that arthritis is a natural part of growing older and that once one gets it, it only gets worse.[5] A study of nursing home residents found that many participants strongly endorsed the belief that there is little potential to improve outcomes with treatment once persistent pain develops.[6] Older adults with pain can also harbor beliefs regarding specific drug and nondrug treatments. Reluctance to take pain medications (particularly opioids) because of a fear of addiction appears to be prevalent.[7] In addition, some older adults believe that use of pain medication will invariably lead to adverse effects.[8] These beliefs may be held by older patients' caregivers who voice reluctance about initiating a course of analgesic medication for their loved one.[9] Research also suggests that many older adults believe that exercise and/or physical activity can hasten disease progression or exacerbate pain.[10–12] **Box 1** lists beliefs endorsed by older adults with pain problems.

Although less research has evaluated the impact of pain-related beliefs on health behaviors, it stands to reason that older adults who believe a given treatment will lead to adverse outcomes, hasten disease progression, or fail to lower pain or improve function will be less likely to try and/or adhere with it over time. Data supporting this hypothesis come from a variety of sources, including a Spanish study that evaluated older adults with chronic pain and assessed for associations between specific pain attitudes and the degree of pain-related interference with everyday life.[13] Participants who strongly endorsed the belief that pain is a signal that damage is occurring were much more likely to report that physical activity should be avoided. In a study of nonelderly adults with chronic pain, researchers evaluated the relationship between specific pain beliefs and medication adherence behaviors.[14] Those who endorsed strong concerns about adverse effects from pain medications and the potential for addiction were much more likely to underuse pain medications. Qualitative research has identified that certain beliefs—uncertainty about the role of exercise as therapy for knee pain or whether exercise can slow disease progression—likely deter individuals from exercising as a form of treatment for their pain.[15] Finally, in 1 study of

---

**Box 1**
**Beliefs and attitudes about pain and pain treatments**

*About Pain*

Pain is a natural part of the aging process

Once one gets it, it only gets worse

People should expect to live with pain when they get older

Chronic pain will not get better even with treatment

It is better to persevere (and live) with pain than seek treatment for it

Complaining about pain could lead to one being labeled a bad patient

*About Pain Treatments*

Pain medications are addictive

Pain medications cause dangerous adverse effects and should be avoided unless absolutely necessary

Pain medications will stop working if taken regularly and lead to the need to take increasing amounts over time

Exercise/physical activity hastens arthritis progression

Avoiding exercise/physical activity is a good way to minimize pain

community-dwelling older adults, participants who endorsed the belief that nothing could be done about their arthritis condition were significantly less likely to have a regular physician, suggesting a relationship between a fatalistic belief and willingness to utilize health resources.[4]

If certain pain beliefs lead to specific behaviors (eg, nonadherence with pain medication, unwillingness to try an exercise program, reluctance/refusal to undergo a needed joint replacement), a key question is whether these beliefs are modifiable. Negative beliefs about the value of exercise were amenable to change in 1 study of exercise for older adults with knee pain and judged to be an important mediator of treatment success.[15] Fear-avoidance beliefs (ie, a worry/concern that physical activities will bring on [or aggravate existing] pain or harm an affected body part) are common in many populations with chronic pain and constitute an important target for intervention efforts. In a small study conducted in a primary care setting, patients with chronic low back pain who received a brief intervention consisting of education and a speed walking task to overcome their fear of movement combined with feedback about their performance endorsed fewer fear-avoidance beliefs following the intervention.[16] A longitudinal study of patients with chronic pain examined the relationships between changes in pain beliefs with change in overall functioning following multidisciplinary treatment.[17] Participants whose belief in their ability to effectively control pain decreased over time were more likely to experience greater disability at a 12-month follow-up after completing treatment. Finally, another study found that decreases in catastrophizing beliefs about pain were associated with less pain-related disability and pain intensity over time.[18]

### Targeting Patient Attitudes and Beliefs in Practice

Existing research supports the notion that certain pain beliefs and attitudes negatively impact older adults' willingness to engage in and/or adhere with treatment, can adversely affect treatment outcomes, and are amenable to change. Clinicians caring for older adults with chronic pain are strongly encouraged to assess patients' beliefs and attitudes prior to initiating any treatment plan and when nonadherence with a treatment is acknowledged by the patient or suspected by the clinician. Existing tools designed to measure patients' beliefs and attitudes about pain (eg, Survey of Pain Attitudes,[19] Pain Belief Questionnaire[20]) and pain treatments (eg, Pain Medication Attitude Questionnaire[14]) are not practical for use in a busy office setting. Open-ended questions (**Box 2**) may be useful and help to elicit erroneous beliefs and attitudes maintained by older patients and their caregivers. Countering erroneous beliefs with

---

**Box 2**
**Questions to ask concerning beliefs and attitudes about pain and pain treatments**

Do you have any beliefs about pain that you think would be important for me to know about?

Do you have any concerns about your pain that are particularly important for me to know about?

Do you have any beliefs about pain that influence your decision making about whether to try or continue to employ a specific pain treatment?

Do you have any beliefs or thoughts about pain treatments that you think it would be important for me to know about?

Do you have any concerns about the treatments you are currently using to help you manage your pain?

simple education often suffices (eg, stating that exercise does not hasten disease progression in patients with arthritis). It may also help patients to point out how a given belief impacts pain (eg, fear of medication adverse effects leads to medication nonadherence, which leads to poorly controlled pain). Some beliefs are harder to counter than others, particularly if the belief has been present for years or is reinforced by others such as the patient's health care provider or caregiver. For these patients, referral to practitioners skilled in delivering cognitive behavioral therapy (CBT) can be helpful, given that challenging unhelpful pain beliefs and changing them constitute core components of CBT.

## PATIENT EXPECTATIONS

Treatment expectancy refers to improvements that patients believe are likely to occur with treatment. Prior research has documented that pretreatment expectations are associated with enhanced treatment outcomes in patients with pain.[21–24] In 1 study of adults receiving CBT for chronic pain, patients who believed that the treatment would help them to cope more effectively with their pain reported enhanced pain coping skills and efficacy for controlling pain at treatment completion and at a 12-month follow-up evaluation.[21] Similar findings have been reported in a large study involving patients with chronic pain receiving multidisciplinary treatment, which found that pretreatment expectations were strong predictors of degree of pain relief and improvement in quality of life.[22] Similar findings have been reported in studies examining acupuncture[23] and treatment for individuals with acute low back pain.[24] These relationships have not been found across all studies. Pretreatment expectations did not predict outcomes among patients undergoing total hip or knee arthroplasty[25] or those receiving acupuncture for chronic low back pain.[26]

Collectively, these data support the notion that for many patients with pain, a more positive outlook regarding the anticipated outcome of therapy (endorsed prior to initiating the trial) can enhance treatment outcomes. Although the mechanisms underlying this effect are not known, possible explanations include enhanced adherence with the therapy among individuals with positive treatment expectations, a placebo effect, adoption of a more positive attitude about their condition, and reporting bias (ie, those who expect enhanced outcomes report improvements to remain consistent in their responses). Treatment expectancies are particularly relevant in the care of older adults with chronic pain, because many affected individuals have undergone multiple failed attempts to treat their pain in the past. Older patients are often unwilling to retry a therapy that provided no benefit in the past. Indeed, many older adults with a history of multiple failed trials find it difficult to believe that meaningful pain relief is achievable (ie, low pre-treatment expectancy). Negative treatment expectations that occur as a consequence of failed analgesic trials in the past have been shown to significantly reduce analgesic efficacy in experimental studies.[27,28] Providers and patients should guard against therapeutic nihilism (ie, the conviction that further treatments are not likely to yield benefit). Clinicians also encounter older patients whose treatment expectations are unrealistically high (eg, "I expect the treatment to make my pain go away entirely"). These patients are challenging, because complete pain eradication is not often possible to achieve.

If patient expectations impact treatment outcomes, are they modifiable? In 1 study of patients undergoing total hip or knee arthroplasty, a simple educational intervention delivered preoperatively was found to change participants' pretreatment expectations regarding outcomes after surgery.[29] Fostering realistic expectations prior to the time of surgery is important, because participants whose expectations are met are more likely to adhere with postoperative recommendations and to report satisfaction with surgical outcomes.[29] Other research indicates that patient expectations can be positively influenced when providers employ both cognitive (providing a clear diagnosis and being optimistic about the anticipated outcome of therapy) and emotional (remaining warm, providing reassurance) techniques during the clinical encounter.[30] Motivational interviewing has also been suggested as a method to help patients modify their expectations.[31]

### Targeting Patient Expectations in Practice

Available research supports the idea that patient expectations can impact treatment outcomes and are potentially malleable. Prior to initiating treatment, clinicians caring for older adults with chronic pain are encouraged to assess patients' treatment expectancies (eg, degree of pain relief expected, degree of anticipated functional improvement). There are several validated questionnaires (eg, Credibility/Expectancy Questionnaire[32] and the Stanford Expectations of Treatment Scale [SETS])[33] that are used to identify expectations of individuals participating in clinical trials. Both scales are short enough to be considered for use in the clinical setting. Other options include single-item questions such as "How much do you expect this treatment will relieve your pain?" Response items could include a 0- to 10 scale, in which a 0 represents "no relief at all," and a 10 represents "complete relief of pain." An ordinal word ranking scale can also be employed where scale anchors might range from "not at all" to "the most I could imagine." Because pretreatment expectancy can vary by outcome, ascertaining patients' expectancies should occur for outcomes patients and providers agree constitute important treatment goals (eg, degree of expected pain relief or functional status enhancement or ability to participate in social activities). Established threshold scores for what constitutes low treatment expectancy (or an unrealistically high treatment expectancy) do not currently exist. Health care providers are encouraged to use their own clinical experience in terms of what constitutes an average treatment response (along with the range of responses encountered in similar patients) to identify older patients whose treatment expectancies are either too low (ie, they do not expect any success) or too high (eg, they expect complete pain relief). Health care providers should educate older patients whose treatment expectancies are very low about what is possible to achieve with the intended therapy. Motivational interviewing may help to change patients' pretreatment expectations that are unrealistically low.[34] Working to instill a hopeful mindset justified by an adequate evidence base is also recommended.[1] Finally, fostering realistic treatment expectations through education is particularly important to do in patients whose treatment expectancies are unrealistically high (and often requires multiple visits).

## PLEASURABLE ACTIVITY SCHEDULING

Many older adults with chronic pain cut back (or eliminate altogether) activities that bring pleasure or meaning to their lives citing chronic pain as a reason.[35] This can include participating in social events, traveling, or pursuing hobbies or recreational activities.[35] Reducing or eliminating pleasurable activities may also occur because of depressed mood and lack of motivation that occur as a consequence of living with chronic pain. Pleasant activity scheduling constitutes a core behavioral coping skill that is present in standard CBT protocols for patients with pain. Patients work with therapists to identify pleasurable/meaningful pursuits, develop a plan to participate in them on a regular basis and work to identify barriers that might get in the way of achieving success. Patients can select unrealistic pursuits at first, so selecting activities that are feasible to accomplish given a patient's functional ability is important to do.

Participating in pleasurable activities is associated with reduced pain.[36,37] The mechanism underlying this effect remains unclear. It may occur because of improved mood or because participating in activities that bring pleasure or meaning successfully distracts patients from their pain, reinforcing the adage that "an occupied mind is the best analgesic."

### Targeting Pleasurable Activity Scheduling in Practice

A large body of literature documents that pleasurable activity restriction is common in patients with chronic pain, associated with decreased quality of life and depressed mood, and can be modified using simple approaches.[35–37] Clinicians are strongly encouraged to include pleasant activity scheduling as part of their multimodal treatment plan, particularly for those patients who endorse cutting back or eliminating pleasurable activities. Even for older patients who report participating in some activities, encouraging them to do more of these activities (with corresponding goal setting) is recommended. For patients who have difficulty endorsing what activities they find pleasurable, providing a list of general pursuits can be helpful. Attention to amotivation or anhedonia as reasons for not being able to identify pleasurable activities is also warranted. Once a list is generated, clinicians can help patients establish a plan to accomplish a defined number of activities (and time spent conducting each) and to brainstorm problems patients may encounter in implementing the plan as a way of identifying barriers that will need to be overcome. The pleasurable activity should be appropriate for the patient's functional abilities and accessible to him or her. Educating patients about benefits likely to be achieved (eg, reduction in pain, improved mood, and for some activities improved physical functioning) is important to do. To reinforce initiation and maintenance of pleasurable activities, the provider should also consider leveraging social supports in the form of family members, home attendants (if appropriate), and community-based agencies. This may take the form of educating family members or other important members of the patient's social network to reinforce and support the patient's engagement in these activities. Revisiting successes achieved at subsequent office visits (or barriers that prevented success) and reinforcing positive results achieved are also important to do.

### SUMMARY

Given the many established barriers to treating pain in older adults, clinicians must seek out additional targets for intervention efforts. Given their impact on treatment outcomes and malleability, clinicians should strongly consider directing their attention to older patients' attitudes and beliefs about pain and pain treatments, expectations regarding treatment outcomes, and pleasurable activity pursuits using practical approaches as described previously. Broadening the portfolio of pain management targets will not guarantee success but enhances the odds of achieving it in this growing population of patients.

### REFERENCES

1. Makris UE, Abrams RC, Gurland B, et al. Management of persistent pain in the older patient: a clinical review. JAMA 2014;312(8):825–36.
2. Reid MC, Eccleston C, Pillemer K. Chronic pain in older adults. BMJ 2015;350: h532.

3. Bandura A. Health promotion by social cognitive means. Health Educ Behav 2004;31:143–64.
4. Goodwin JS, Black SA, Satish S. Aging versus disease: the opinions of older black, Hispanic, and non-Hispanic-white Americans about the causes and treatment of common medical conditions. J Am Geriatr Soc 1999;47:973–9.
5. Appelt CJ, Burant CJ, Siminoff LA, et al. Arthritis-specific health beliefs related to aging among older male patients with knee and/or hip osteoarthritis. J Gerontol A Biol Sci Med Sci 2007;62(2):184–90.
6. Weiner DK, Rudy TE. Attitudinal barriers to effective treatment of persistent pain in nursing home residents. J Am Geriatr Soc 2003;50:2035–40.
7. Auret K, Schug SA. Underutilization of opioids in elderly patients with chronic pain: APPROACHES to correcting the problem. Drugs Aging 2005;22(8):641–54.
8. Gunnarsdottir S, Donovan HS, Serline RC, et al. Patient-related barriers to pain management: the barriers questionnaire II (BQ-II). Pain 2002;99(3):385–96.
9. Spitz A, Moore AA, Papaleontiou M, et al. Primary care providers' perspective on prescribing opioids to older adults with chronic non-cancer pain: a qualitative study. BMC Geriatr 2011;11:35.
10. Marks R, Allegrante JP. Chronic osteoarthritis and adherence to exercise: a review of the literature. J Aging Phys Act 2005;13:434–60.
11. Hendry M, Williams NH, Markland D, et al. Why should we exercise when our knees hurt? A qualitative study of primary care patients with osteoarthritis of the knee. Fam Pract 2006;23(5):558–67.
12. Holden MA, Nicholls EE, Young J, et al. Role of exercise for knee pain: what do older adults in the community think? Arthritis Care Res 2012;64(10):1554–64.
13. Miro J, Queral R, del Carme Nolla M. Pain-related attitudes and functioning in elderly primary care patients. Span J Psychol 2014;17:E104.
14. McCracken LM, Hoskins J, Eccleston C. Concerns about medication and medication use in chronic pain. J Pain 2006;7(10):726–34.
15. Hurley MV, Walsh N, Bhavnani V, et al. Health beliefs before and after participation on an exercise-based rehabilitation programme for chronic knee pain: doing is believing. BMC Musculoskelet Disord 2010;11:31.
16. Guck TP, Burke RV, Rainville C, et al. A brief primary care intervention to reduce fear of movement in chronic low back pain patients. Transl Behav Med 2015;5(1):113–21.
17. Jensen MP, Turner JA, Romano JM. Changes after multidisciplinary pain treatment in patient pain beliefs and coping are associated with concurrent changes in patient functioning. Pain 2007;131(1–2):38–47.
18. Jensen MP, Turner JA, Romano JM. Changes in beliefs, catastrophizing, and coping are associated with improvement in multidisciplinary treatment. J Consult Clin Psychol 2001;69(4):655–62.
19. Jensen MP, Karoly P, Huger R. The development and preliminary validation of an instrument to assess patients' attitudes toward pain. J Psychosom Res 1987;31:393–400.
20. Edwards LC, Pearce SA, Turner-Stokes L, et al. The pain beliefs questionnaire: an investigation of beliefs in the causes and consequences of pain. Pain 1992;51:267–72.
21. Goosens MEJB, Vlaeyen JWS, Hidding A, et al. Treatment expectancy affects the outcome of cognitive-behavioral interventions in chronic pain. Clin J Pain 2005;21(1):18–26.
22. Cormier S, Lavigne GL, Choiniere M, et al. Expectations predict chronic pain treatment outcomes. Pain 2016;157(2):329–38.

23. Linde K, Witt CM, Streng A, et al. The impact of patient expectations on outcomes in four randomized controlled trials of acupuncture in patients with chronic pain. Pain 2007;128:264–71.

24. Myers SS, Phillips RS, Davis RB, et al. Patient expectations as predictors of outcome in patients with acute low back pain. J Gen Intern Med 2007;23(2): 148–53.

25. Haanstra TM, van den Berg T, Ostelo RW, et al. Systematic revew: do patient expectations influence treatment outcomes in total knee and total hip arthroplasty? Health Qual Life Outcomes 2012;10:152.

26. Sherman KJ, Cherkin DC, Ichikawa L, et al. Treatment expectations and preferences of outcome of acupuncture for chronic back pain. Spine 2010;35(15): 1471–7.

27. Bingel U, Wanigasekera V, Wiech K, et al. The effect of treatment expectation on drug efficacy: imaging the analgesic benefit of the opioid remifentanil. Sci Transl Med 2011;3(70):70ra14.

28. Kessner S, Wiech K, Forkmann K, et al. The effect of treatment history on therapeutic outcome; an experimental approach. JAMA Intern Med 2013;173(15): 1468–9.

29. Mancuso CA, Graziano S, Briskie LM. Randomized trials to modify patients' preoperative expectations of hip and knee arthroplasties. Clin Orthop Relat Res 2008;466:424–31.

30. Blasi ZD, Harkness E, Ernst E, et al. Influence of context effects on health outcomes: a systematic review. Lancet 2001;357:757–62.

31. Werstra HA. Motivational Interviewing in the treatment of anxiety. New York: Guilford Press; 2015.

32. Devilly GJ, Borkovec TD. Psychometric properties of the credibility/expectancy questionnaire. J Behav Ther Exp Psychiatry 2000;31:73–86.

33. Younger J, Gandhi V, Hubbard E, et al. Development of the Stanford Expectations Treatment Scale (SETS): a tool for measuring patient outcome expectancy in clinical trials. Clin Trials 2012;9:767–76.

34. Broderick JE, Junghaenel DU, Schneider S, et al. Treatment expectations for pain coping skills training: relationship to osteoarthritis patients' baseline psychosocial characteristics. Clin J Pain 2011;27(4):315–22.

35. Duong BD, Kerns RD, Reid MC. Identifying the activities affected by chronic pain in older persons. J Am Geriatr Soc 2005;53:687–94.

36. Murphy JL, McKellar JD, Raffa SD, et al. Cognitive behavioral therapy for chronic pain: therapist manual. Washington, DC: U.S. Department of Veterans Affairs; 2014.

37. Keefe FJ, Kashikar-Zuck S, Opiteck J, et al. Pain in arthritis and musculoskeletal disorders: the role of coping skills training and exercise interventions. J Orthop Sports Phys Ther 1996;24(4):279–90.

# Index

*Note:* Page numbers of article titles are in **boldface** type.

Clin Geriatr Med 32 (2016) 807–811
http://dx.doi.org/10.1016/S0749-0690(16)30090-8
0749-0690/16/$ – see front matter

geriatric.theclinics.com

# UNITED STATES POSTAL SERVICE® Statement of Ownership, Management, and Circulation
## (All Periodicals Publications Except Requester Publications)

| 1. Publication Title | 2. Publication Number | 3. Filing Date |
|---|---|---|
| CLINICS IN GERIATRIC MEDICINE | 000 – 704 | 9/18/2016 |

| 4. Issue Frequency | 5. Number of Issues Published Annually | 6. Annual Subscription Price |
|---|---|---|
| FEB, MAY, AUG, NOV | 4 | $269.00 |

7. Complete Mailing Address of Known Office of Publication (Not printer) (Street, city, county, state, and ZIP+4®)

ELSEVIER INC.
360 PARK AVENUE SOUTH
NEW YORK, NY 10010-1710

Contact Person
STEPHEN R. BUSHING

Telephone (Include area code)
215-239-3688

8. Complete Mailing Address of Headquarters or General Business Office of Publisher (Not printer)

ELSEVIER INC.
360 PARK AVENUE SOUTH
NEW YORK, NY 10010-1710

9. Full Names and Complete Mailing Addresses of Publisher, Editor, and Managing Editor (Do not leave blank)

Publisher (Name and complete mailing address)

LINDA BELFUS, ELSEVIER INC.
1600 JOHN F KENNEDY BLVD. SUITE 1800
PHILADELPHIA, PA 19103-2899

Editor (Name and complete mailing address)

JESSICA MCCOOL, ELSEVIER INC.
1600 JOHN F KENNEDY BLVD. SUITE 1800
PHILADELPHIA, PA 19103-2899

Managing Editor (Name and complete mailing address)

ADRIANNE BRIGIDO, ELSEVIER INC.
1600 JOHN F KENNEDY BLVD. SUITE 1800
PHILADELPHIA, PA 19103-2899

10. Owner (Do not leave blank. If the publication is owned by a corporation, give the name and address of the corporation immediately followed by the names and addresses of all stockholders owning or holding 1 percent or more of the total amount of stock. If not owned by a corporation, give the names and addresses of the individual owners. If owned by a partnership or other unincorporated firm, give its name and address as well as those of each individual owner. If the publication is published by a nonprofit organization, give its name and address.)

| Full Name | Complete Mailing Address |
|---|---|
| WHOLLY OWNED SUBSIDIARY OF REED/ELSEVIER, US HOLDINGS | 1600 JOHN F KENNEDY BLVD. SUITE 1800 PHILADELPHIA, PA 19103-2899 |

11. Known Bondholders, Mortgagees, and Other Security Holders Owning or Holding 1 Percent or More of Total Amount of Bonds, Mortgages, or Other Securities. If none, check box ▶ ☐ None

| Full Name | Complete Mailing Address |
|---|---|
| N/A | |

12. Tax Status (For completion by nonprofit organizations authorized to mail at nonprofit rates) (Check one)
The purpose, function, and nonprofit status of this organization and the exempt status for federal income tax purposes:
☐ Has Not Changed During Preceding 12 Months
☐ Has Changed During Preceding 12 Months (Publisher must submit explanation of change with this statement)

| 13. Publication Title | 14. Issue Date for Circulation Data Below |
|---|---|
| CLINICS IN GERIATRIC MEDICINE | AUGUST 2016 |

| 15. Extent and Nature of Circulation | | Average No. Copies Each Issue During Preceding 12 Months | No. Copies of Single Issue Published Nearest to Filing Date |
|---|---|---|---|
| a. Total Number of Copies (Net press run) | | 276 | 327 |
| b. Paid Circulation (By Mail and Outside the Mail) | (1) Mailed Outside-County Paid Subscriptions Stated on PS Form 3541 (Include paid distribution above nominal rate, advertiser's proof copies, and exchange copies) | 96 | 117 |
| | (2) Mailed In-County Paid Subscriptions Stated on PS Form 3541 (Include paid distribution above nominal rate, advertiser's proof copies, and exchange copies) | 0 | 0 |
| | (3) Paid Distribution Outside the Mails Including Sales Through Dealers and Carriers, Street Vendors, Counter Sales, and Other Paid Distribution Outside USPS® | 61 | 77 |
| | (4) Paid Distribution by Other Classes of Mail Through the USPS (e.g., First-Class Mail®) | 0 | 0 |
| c. Total Paid Distribution [Sum of 15b (1), (2), (3), and (4)] | ▶ | 157 | 194 |
| d. Free or Nominal Rate Distribution (By Mail and Outside the Mail) | (1) Free or Nominal Rate Outside-County Copies included on PS Form 3541 | 48 | 68 |
| | (2) Free or Nominal Rate In-County Copies included on PS Form 3541 | 0 | 0 |
| | (3) Free or Nominal Rate Copies Mailed at Other Classes Through the USPS (e.g., First-Class Mail) | 0 | 0 |
| | (4) Free or Nominal Rate Distribution Outside the Mail (Carriers or other means) | 0 | 0 |
| e. Total Free or Nominal Rate Distribution (Sum of 15d (1), (2), (3) and (4)) | ▶ | 48 | 68 |
| f. Total Distribution (Sum of 15c and 15e) | ▶ | 205 | 262 |
| g. Copies not Distributed (See Instructions to Publishers #4 (page #3)) | ▶ | 71 | 65 |
| h. Total (Sum of 15f and g) | ▶ | 276 | 327 |
| i. Percent Paid (15c divided by 15f times 100) | ▶ | 77% | 74% |

* If you are claiming electronic copies, go to line 16 on page 3. If you are not claiming electronic copies, skip to line 17 on page 3.

| 16. Electronic Copy Circulation | Average No. Copies Each Issue During Preceding 12 Months | No. Copies of Single Issue Published Nearest to Filing Date |
|---|---|---|
| a. Paid Electronic Copies ▶ | 0 | 0 |
| b. Total Paid Print Copies (Line 15c) + Paid Electronic Copies (Line 16a) ▶ | 157 | 194 |
| c. Total Print Distribution (Line 15f) + Paid Electronic Copies (Line 16a) ▶ | 205 | 262 |
| d. Percent Paid (Both Print & Electronic Copies) (16b divided by 16c × 100) ▶ | 77% | 74% |

☒ I certify that 50% of all my distributed copies (electronic and print) are paid above a nominal price.

17. Publication of Statement of Ownership
☒ If the publication is a general publication, publication of this statement is required. Will be printed ☐ Publication not required.
in the NOVEMBER 2016 issue of this publication.

18. Signature and Title of Editor, Publisher, Business Manager, or Owner

STEPHEN R. BUSHING - INVENTORY DISTRIBUTION CONTROL MANAGER

Date 9/18/2016

I certify that all information furnished on this form is true and complete. I understand that anyone who furnishes false or misleading information on this form or who omits material or information requested on the form may be subject to criminal sanctions (including fines and imprisonment) and/or civil sanctions (including civil penalties).

PS Form 3526, July 2014 (Page 3 of 4)

PRIVACY NOTICE: See our privacy policy on www.usps.com.

Printed and bound by CPI Group (UK) Ltd, Croydon, CR0 4YY

03/10/2024

01040397-0019